SPECTACULAR SEX MOVES

she'll NEVER FORGET

INGENIOUS POSITIONS AND TECHNIQUES
THAT WILL BLOW HER MIND

Text © 2010 Sonia Borg, Ph.D., M.A., M.P.H.
Photography © 2011 Quiver

First published in the USA in 2011 by
Quiver, a member of
Quayside Publishing Group
100 Cummings Center
Suite 406-L
Beverly, MA 01915-6101
www.quiverbooks.com

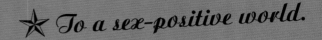
To a sex-positive world.

The publisher maintains the records relating to images in this book required by 18 USC 2257. Records are
located at Rockport Publishers, Inc., 100 Cummings Center, Suite 406-L, Beverly, MA 01915-6101.

A Note to Readers:
This book contains the opinions and ideas of the author and is intended for the use of informed and
consenting adults. It's not therapy; it's fun.

Sonia Borg, Ph.D., M.P.H. is a clinical sexologist and a sex coach, not a therapist or medical doctor. Some
of the practices and positions in this book may not be appropriate for people with medical conditions or
physical impairments. Use your good judgment!

ISBN-13: 978-1-59233-480-3
ISBN-10: 1-59233-480-6

Library of Congress Cataloging-in-Publication Data is available

Book design by Holtz Design
Photography by Holly Randall
Illustrations by Robert Brandt

Printed and bound in Singapore

SONIA BORG PH.D. , M.A., M.P.H.
AUTHOR OF *ORAL SEX SHE'LL NEVER FORGET*

SPECTACULAR SEX MOVES
she'll NEVER FORGET

INGENIOUS POSITIONS AND TECHNIQUES
THAT WILL BLOW HER MIND

QUIVER

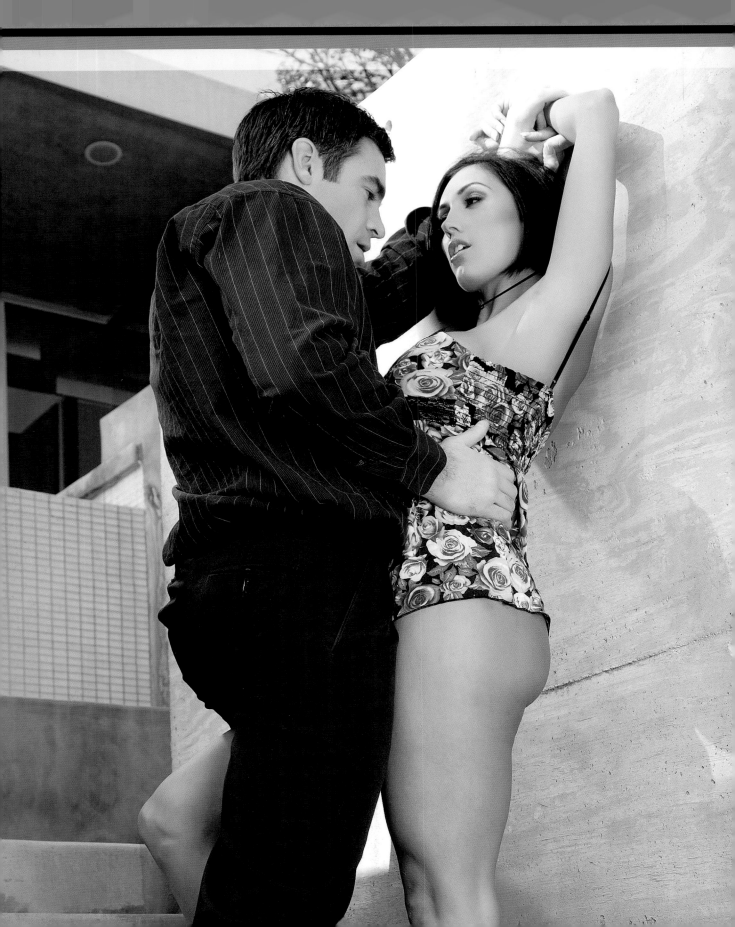

Contents

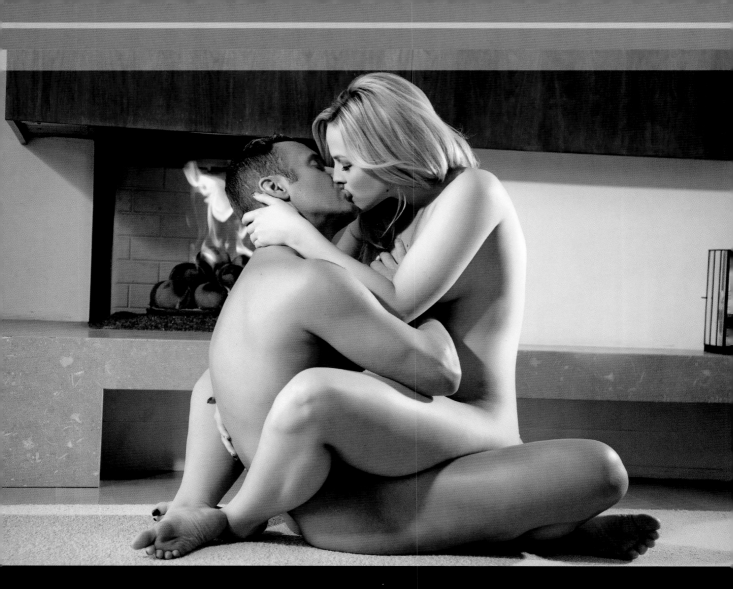

 # INTRODUCTION

This book will teach you how to move and navigate with a woman to total and complete sexual satisfaction (hers and yours). In the process you will discover increased confidence in your own skills as a lover; energy and empowerment via a new form of communication; a newly inspired sense of sexual adventure and creativity; and a sense of freedom derived from living outside your comfort zone.

I promise both you and your lover this: your relationship will feel new and exciting again.

The book is organized into different sections so you can master positioning quickly and easily:

- ★ He's on Top
- ★ She's on Top
- ★ Rear Entry
- ★ Sitting and Kneeling
- ★ Standing
- ★ Side by Side
- ★ Oral Sex
- ★ Hand Jobs
- ★ Moregasms

Other books may teach you different position techniques, but this book does more than that: I have created a series of erotic scenarios for every mood to turn sex into an event. Each exciting and creative scenario helps you master positioning and includes step-by-step segments for foolproof erotic play. The Preparations give you all the little preparatory details while The Lead-In guides you through the first step and helps initiate the act. The Foreplay lays down a unique and appropriate warm-up, and The Main Act gives you step-by-step directions to reach orgasm. Simply put, you will always know what to do next.

I've also included several other types of material, such as Why It Works for Her and Why It Works for Him. These sections explain the "why" behind the move, multiplying your sexual knowledge and increasing your sexual satisfaction. I've also sprinkled Sex Facts throughout the book to boost your sexual prowess, and The Sexpert Says sections give you useful information based on my own experience, observations as a clinical sexologist, and confessions from clients. The notes here will help you understand how to be creative, light, and playful with sex; provide a snapshot of female sexuality; and give you some insight into male sexuality, too.

There is an erotic scenario here for every mood, from playful to soul mate connection. If you try one and don't like it, try another . . . and another . . . and another. Adapt, change, and modify to make each scenario your own. Don't worry about doing the positions and techniques properly. Practice the techniques, do them, and then forget about them. Find your own sense of freedom and creativity, and most important, have fun.

I sincerely hope that my book will give you the tools and inspiration for rocking her erotic world.

Wishing you a healthy and happy sex life!
xoxox,

Dr. Sonia

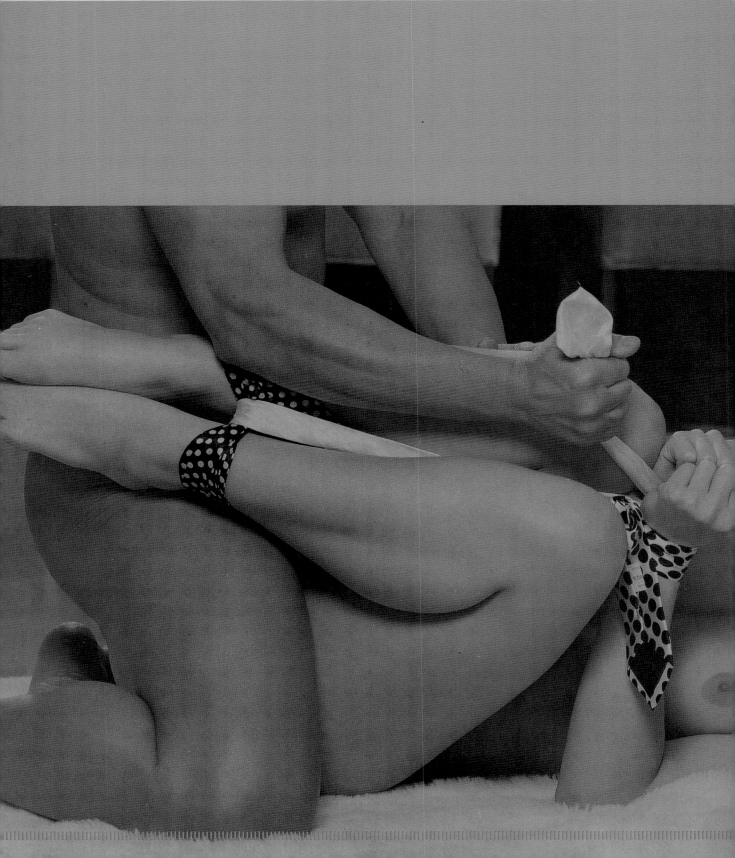

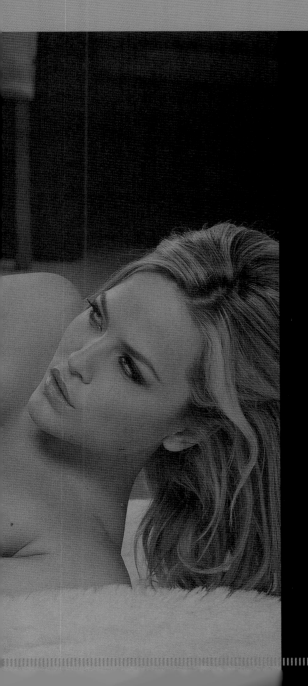

He's On Top

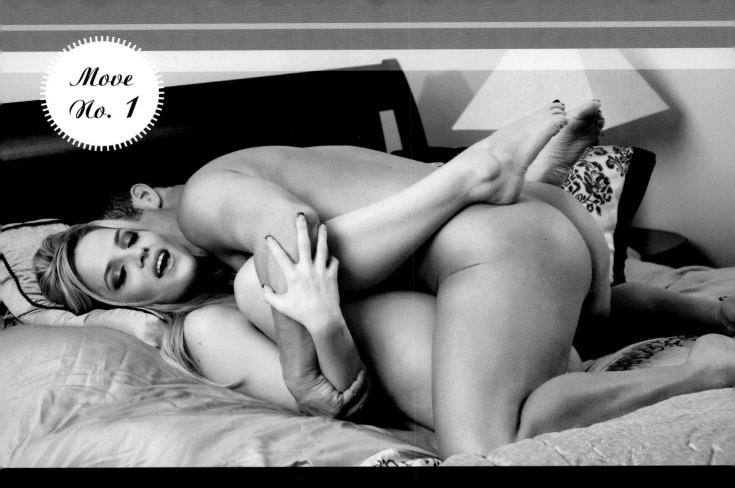

 # CLITTY CAT
(Coital Alignment Technique)

Imagine for a moment the alignment of your bodies during missionary sex. Depending on your physical body sizes, she may or may not be getting the clitoral stimulation that will help her climax. To help us all become more conscious of this, hard-working sex researchers came up with a technique called Coital Alignment Technique. Women who used this method reported a 56 percent increase in orgasm during sex. This scenario will teach you the move, how it works, why it is so effective, and some thrilling variations to spice it up.

The Move: Clitty Cat

THE PREPARATIONS

★ Men and women are inclined to do what feels best during sex. Clap your hands together for a moment. Generally speaking, the quick insertion and removal that offers a full stroke to the cock is the kind of thrust a man generally gravitates to during intercourse. In fact, you can often hear a clapping sound during man-on-top intercourse. Now rub your hands together slowly. This is an example of the type of thrusting that a woman typically gravitates to during intercourse because there is constant rubbing on her clitoris.

★ The Clitty Cat works because of the alignment with and stimulation to the clitoris. In this scenario, you want to visualize the clit, see the clit, and be the clit. Imagine yourself in the missionary position rubbing, grinding, and bumping her clitoris on your penis, the place where your pubic bone meets the base of your penis. Review Xtra Mileage on page 140, so you can learn techniques for better control and lasting longer. All things considered, men generally take less time to orgasm than women do.

★ Do you shave? Shave your balls and leave the hair on the pubic bone trimmed or fluffy soft for nice clit rubbing. Trimming the scrotum makes your penis appear larger, increases sensation to your balls, and is more oral sex–friendly because she will be able to glide a tongue over a smooth surface. Leaving your pubic bone fluffy or trimmed provides a nice pillow for the clitoris. Remember, there are more than 8,000 nerve endings in the clitoris. Stubbles happen with shaving and when it does, she may *avoid* the rubbing to her clit that can help bring her to orgasm. Alternatively, you could always wax.

★ Shave your face so your whiskers don't irritate her delicate skin.

★ Practice the downward thrust on the edge of a horizontally placed pillow, pretending the edge of the pillow is her clit.

THE LEAD-IN

Give her a copy of my book, *Spectacular Sex Moves He'll Never Forget* (trust me, you will be happy you did). Write a note that says, "I am reading *Spectacular Sex Moves She'll Never Forget*. Let's choose one chapter each and do it tonight."

Place the note inside the book so it is hanging out and clearly visible. Wrap the sexy book and leave it for her to open before she leaves the house. This could be a great way to suggest many more sexcapades in the future.

||||||||||||||||||||||||||||||||||||||||||||||||||||||||||||||||||||||||||||||||||||||||||||||||||||||||||||||

SEX FACT

According to a survey by MSNBC/*Elle* magazine, the best predictors of sexual satisfaction for women are deep kissing, gentle kissing, and changing positions. For men, it is changing sexual positions, receiving oral sex, and deep kissing (in that order).

THE FOREPLAY

① Let's help make sure that everyone is sexually satisfied by doing it all: deep kissing, gentle kissing, oral sex, and changing positions.

② Get up close to your lover with lips almost touching and eyes closed, and gently graze the surface of her mouth. Allow yourself to get lost in the kiss. If your mind wanders, bring it back and feel the lip-to-lip sensation, listen to her breath, and smell her scent.

③ Enter into deep kissing with the tip of your tongue on her lips and inside her mouth (never insert your full tongue). Circle her tongue with yours and pull back in a rhythmic fashion as you caress her face and stroke her hair. Make eye contact while you open her shirt, then use your tongue to explore your way down to her neck, shoulders, and breasts. Kiss and flick your tongue on each of her nipples. Kiss your way down to her waist and tongue along the waistband of her panties; when you are ready, slowly remove them with your teeth.

④ Go for oral. Lay her down on the bed while you lie down in the opposite direction in the form of a 69 position with each of your topmost legs bent and your feet flat for easy access to each other's genitals. You can rest your head on the bed or use each other's flat leg as a pillow. Notice your energy move and magnify.

⑤ Wrap your arms around her and spread her butt cheeks open. Pull your head back slightly so you can lay a flat tongue over her clitoris and move your face from side to side, pressing your nose on her perineum and running your fingers over her anus. Move just the tip of your tongue sideways over the commissure and then gently rub your tongue up and down the shaft of her clit to the tip; occasionally, lightly brush over the clitoral gland and suck. Repeat.

||||||||||||||||||||||||||||||||||||||||||||||||||||||||||||||||||||||||||||||||||||||||||||||||||||||||||||||

THE SEXPERT SAYS

There are many reasons why a woman does not climax during intercourse, but teaching her to rub her clitoris is the first place to start. Also, try adopting the two-to-one philosophy: that is, she gets two orgasms for every one of yours. Many women do not need to go through the entire sexual response cycle for another climax. They are in a high arousal state after the first.

⭐ The Main Act

1 Move onto your knees and lean over her; she can wrap her legs around or just below your buttocks. Position your erection so the pubic bone of your penis is pressing against her clitoris.

2 Now for the rhythmic thrusts. Move slowly and try to keep your pubic bone pressed against her clitoris at all times as you penetrate her; move in opposing rocking thrusts. You will be moving your pelvis downward during the inward stroke, and upward for the outward stroke.

3 Find her rhythm and expand on it. Encourage her to raise her pelvis and thrust, or show her by leaning to one side and putting your hand under her rear as you lift her bum and press it against your pubic bone.

4 Continue to move slowly, but don't forget to get feedback and ask her what feels good. When you get the motion, or just the right spot, have her tell you so.

5 The consistent sexual movement in all the right spots builds arousal that peaks naturally. Find your rhythm and groove as you rub and tickle the Clitty Cat all the way to orgasm.

RELATED MOVES

★ Crossing her legs over your rear helps her pull herself up and rub her clit against you. Alternatively, you can place pillows under her lower back to shorten the distance and make upward thrusting easier for her. Spreading or opening her legs can make for deeper penetration.

★ This move takes practice with a partner. If you put it aside in favor of a more familiar position, pick it up again another time with more mindfulness.

♀ WHY IT WORKS FOR HER

★ Her "clitty cat" will be nice and sated with the vaginal and clitoral sensations and possibly intensify and multiply her orgasms.

★ If she didn't already know to thrust and rub her clit during intercourse before doing the Clitty Cat, she does now, and that is an incredible gift.

♂ WHY IT WORKS FOR HIM

★ You will learn a new position and a technique that can increase her chances of orgasm.

★ You'll also gain increased awareness of your own bodies and how they work together.

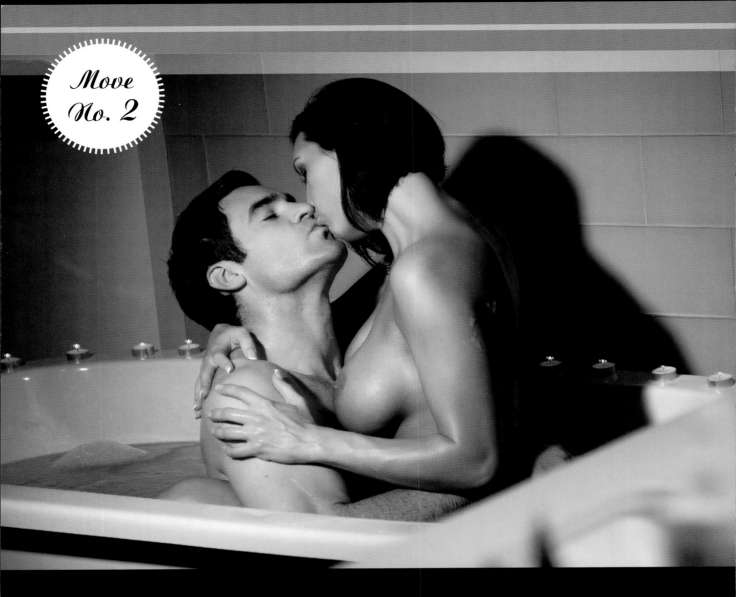

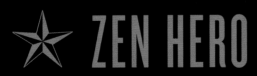 # ZEN HERO

How many times have you had a sexual release so you can relax and go to sleep? One of the greatest gifts that men can give women is their presence and their amazing grounding energies. Many women try to do way too much and the result is always the same—stress. In this scene you are the Zen hero calming her with your rhythmic, rocking penetration.

The Move: Zen Hero

THE PREPARATIONS

Prepare a Zen kit to have on hand, so you can be prepared when the time arises:

- ★ Candles
- ★ Lighter or matches
- ★ Bubble bath
- ★ Relaxing music
- ★ Lavender massage oil/lotions
- ★ Chamomile tea

When the need for nurturing strikes, draw a bath and add bubbles, light the candles, put on the relaxing music, and pour some hot, calming tea.

THE LEAD-IN

As soon as you feel the stressed energy, give her a grounding hug. To start, stand with your legs hip-width apart. Feel the ground underneath your feet. Take a deep breath and fill your belly with air. Exhale and imagine all your cares and concerns disappearing. Keep encouraging her to follow suit, leading her to breathe fuller and deeper. Reach for her hand and put it on your heart. Now, put your hand on her heart and imagine your heart opening as you rock back and forth to your heartbeats into a soothing trance. Lead her to the bubble bath.

THE FOREPLAY

① Undress her slowly and gently, then undress yourself and climb into the tub. Invite her to sit in front of you in the bathtub. Let her lean back onto your chest and let go. Men offer many gifts, but feelings of safety and comfort are among the best.

② Get playful. Move the bubbles to cover her nipples and then playfully blow them off. Play with her hair and push it aside to kiss her neck and ears.

③ Offer to wash her hair, and give her a nice scalp massage at the same time, rubbing the temples and entire surface of the scalp with your fingertips. Follow this by gently pulling her hair, taking her deeper and deeper into relaxation. Scalp massages have many benefits, including the ability to alleviate stress and anxiety. Plus, it just plain feels good to have your hair washed.

④ Get out of the bath first so you can wrap her in a dry towel and hold her in your arms. Walk her to the bed, look her in the eye, and remove her towel so it drops to the floor.

||||||||||||||||||||||||||||||||||||||||||||||||||||||||||||||||||||||||||||||||||||||||||||||||||||||

SEX FACT

According to an MSNBC/*Elle* survey, 42 percent of women say stress is the number one reason they didn't have sex in the last month. (Maybe it should be the reason we *do* have sex!)

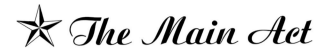 The Main Act

1 Take your rhythm to the bed. Gently lay her down on her back and bend her knees to her chest. Position yourself in front of her, on your knees. Lean forward, holding on to her knees firmly, so she can let go and release. (See above right.)

2 Enter her with a full rock movement, finding the flow. Push your pelvis against hers, rubbing your pubic bone against her clitoris.

3 For G-spot stimulation, aim upward and give a shallow thrust. For more depth and cervix stimulation, aim back with a full thrust.

4 Keep your intention to make love, rocking and moving to the beat. Making love is not about the position, speed, or frequency at which you touch your lover, but about the intention behind the act. As long as the intention is there, you can fuck as fast and hard as you want.

5 Thrust really fast or slow and then just stop, feel, and appreciate all the feelings. Continue the process all the way to orgasm.

6 Spoon her in the fetal position with her knees to her chest while you hold and rock her throughout resolution.

RELATED MOVES

★ Restrain her so she doesn't have to make a single decision about sex.

★ Lift her ankles and shift them from one side of your body to the other. (See below right.) This will continue to rock-roll and release any tension in her pelvis; the motion will cause the vaginal muscles to contract around your penis.

♀ WHY IT WORKS FOR HER

★ She will adore all the nurturing and caring. This position, with her knees to her chest, gives deep penetration toward her cervix.

♂ WHY IT WORKS FOR HIM

★ By its nature, this position will allow you to slow down, be in the moment, and last longer. Lasting longer means more pleasure for you and her.

★ The position also engages all of your senses at once: seeing her, feeling her, tasting her, hearing her, and smelling her, which all contribute to intensifying your orgasm.

SEX FACTS

Sex researcher William Reich believes the best way to release the extra energy and built-up tension from the day is sexual orgasm.

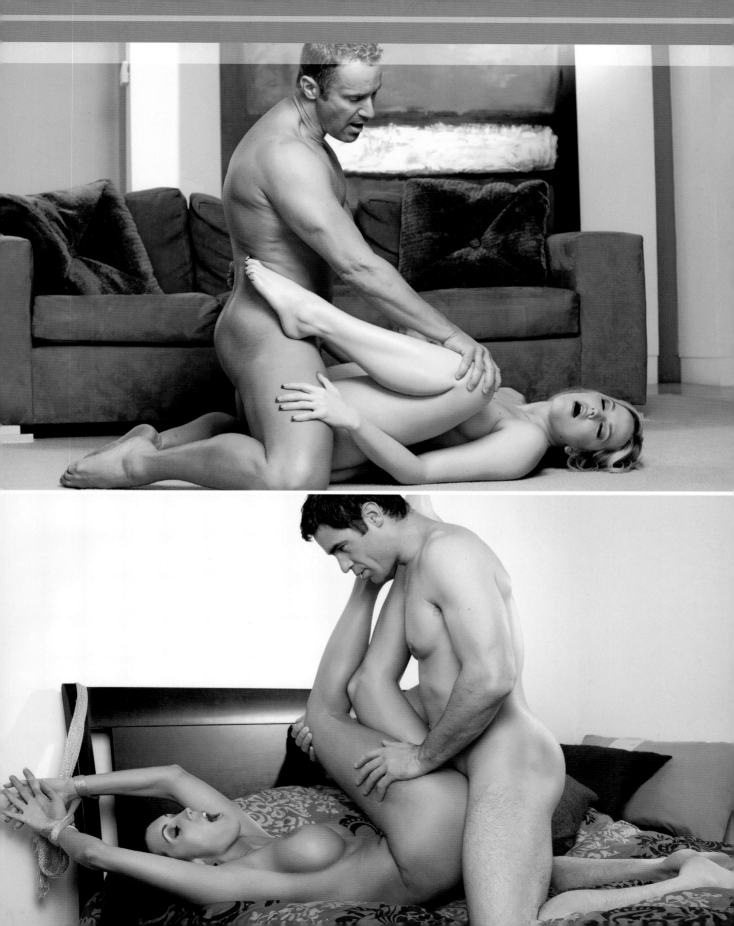

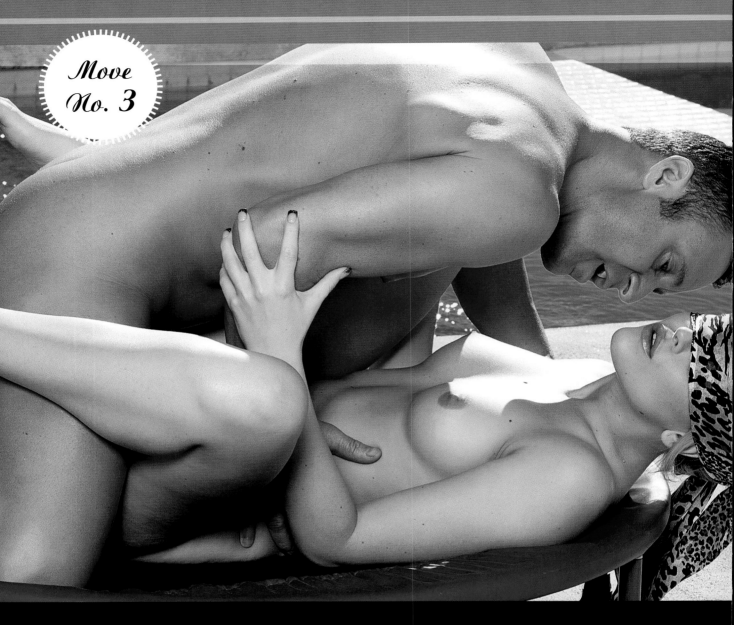

 # BACKYARD BONK

Get naked, get silly, and get on top as you bounce her on your backyard trampoline or adult bouncy house. She will be wild with a sense of freedom and you will get some excellent views of her bouncing breasts and soaring pussy.

The Move: Backyard Bonk

THE PREPARATIONS

★ Rent or buy a new or used large trampoline. Alternatively, bouncy houses are usually readily available for rent and can make a good substitution.

★ Wash the trampoline off and have a towel handy for whoever is on the bottom. Those trampolines can give a nasty burn. Set up the hose and sprinkler.

THE LEAD-IN

Invite her to a happy hour for two, giving her the date and time in advance. Pour her a drink and blindfold her, then lead her to the trampoline or bouncy house. Take off her shoes and help her up. Take off your clothes. Hold her hands and do a few bounces together. When you see a smile break, take off the blindfold and bounce naked with your penis flapping in the air. Now that the apprehension of looking silly is over, invite her to join in. Remove her clothes for her, or ask her to try and take her clothes off while she bounces. Relax, laugh, and get into the fun of it all.

THE FOREPLAY

① If the weather is warm, have a splash and put the sprinkler under the trampoline.

② See who can jump the highest or twirl while jumping. Remember, this isn't a *real* competition, just fun and playful, so support her silliness.

③ Turn it sweet by bouncing together holding hands. Time it right for a kiss in the air.

④ Turn it playful by giving her a couple of slaps on the ass mid-bounce. Ask her to jump up and give you a shot of her beautiful pussy. See if you can caress her nipples or rub her clit while bouncing.

⑤ Slow down the bounce to a stop, place the towel down, and lie her down on the trampoline on her back. Use a pillow for added comfort and depth positioning.

⑥ Spread open her legs and go down to her pussy. Start with a few full coverage strokes with a flat tongue all over her vulva. Then move your head up and down, bouncing your flat tongue on her clit. Gradually point your tongue on the commissure so the pressure becomes centralized.

||||||||||||||||||||||||||||||||||||||||||||||||||||||||||||||||||||||||||||||||||||||||||||||||||||||||||||||||||||||||

SEX FACT

Acrophilia mamaquatia is an erotic fixation with heights and the bobbing of a woman's breasts during exercise.

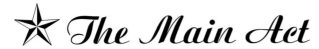 # The Main Act

1 Get on top of her as if in regular missionary style, hands beside her shoulders, and insert your cock. Even though she may be on her back, this is not a passive position and anything but dull.

2 The key is to find your rhythm and timing so you can let the trampoline do most of the work. It's almost like swinging on a swing. Once you get the flow of the swing, you only have to give a good pump once in a while.

3 Keeping your arms steady, start off slowly and use your feet and pelvis to get the rhythm going. Go for depth rather than in and outs. In and outs, especially when adding a new dynamic, can bring about some "misses."

4 Although it feels unusual to have an additional bounce, you are both searching for the pattern, timing, and rhythm that feels good. When you find it, move, groove, ride, bump, pump, and grind to orgasm.

5 Hold her and celebrate this playful event throughout resolution.

6 Save the blindfold. It is great for heightening senses and turning a regular day, or sexual position, into a surprising adventure. Or simply take it out and leave it visible as a reminder of your summer fun.

||||||||||||||||||||||||||||||||||||||||||||||||||||||||||||||||||||||||||||||||||||||||||||||||||||||||||||||||||||||||

SEX FACT

According to a survey by MSNBC/*Elle* magazine, 68 percent of women said their sex life was predictable. (She will not expect this move!)

RELATED MOVES

★ Lie on your back and let her sit on top, facing backward toward your feet. This will allow her to be in control for a bit and give her depth and bounce without your penis coming all the way out.

♀ WHY IT WORKS FOR HER

★ She gets reacquainted with her playful side, and that offers a sense of freedom. Who knows what could happen? She will also enjoy feeling your weight and pressure on her body and the depth of penetration that this position offers.

♂ WHY IT WORKS FOR HIM

★ You are the creativity hero, saving you both from the bedroom boredom that can creep into all of our lives at some point. The extra bounce in this position gives maximum depth of penetration with less effort on your part. And you will love feeling your balls slapping against her ass!

|||||||||||||||||||||||||||||||||||||||||||||||||||||||||||||||||||||||||||||||||||||||||||||||||||||||||||||||||||||||||||||

THE SEXPERT SAYS

It may not come wrapped in a bow, have a membership fee, or be printed on an admission ticket, but that doesn't mean sex is not a gift or a form of exercise, entertainment, adventure, play, and fun. Sex can be all those things and more. Sex is what you make it.

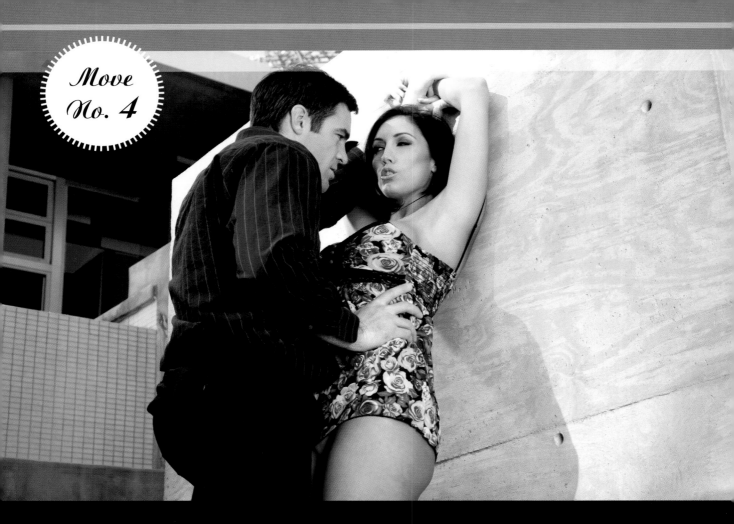

THE ALCHEMIST

Women everywhere got wet between the legs when Rhett from *Gone with the Wind* landed a big kiss on Scarlet, swept her up the stairs, and fucked the bitchiness right out of her. The next time your girl is being a you-know-what, go ahead and call it what it is—being a bitch—and then react in a way she will never expect—with love, playfulness, and sex.

This position satisfies one of the top female fantasies (force) and allows her to have an emotional release, or emotion-gasm, leaving no option to *not* enjoy sex. Lift her arms over her head, spread her legs wide open, and offer resistance and maybe a little spanking from the one who knows what's best for her. Alchemize that bitch energy into solid sex gold and take your passion up about ten notches. Lightness, fun, and play are the secret ways to a woman's heart

The Move: The Alchemist

THE PREPARATIONS

★ It's easy to get into patterns of living and being with our partners, even in regard to arguing. List the different ways you can respond with play, light, ease, and sex. Talk about it with your partner and agree not to sweat the small stuff with sex. I'm talking about the silly things we get caught up in, not the serious stuff. You may want to consider sharing this scenario and coming to an agreement to do it when the time is right.

★ It's more about the energy and intention than the act. One of the best sexual skills you can have is knowing how to read your partner's energy. Men and women want and need different things at different times, and that includes sex. Sometimes we want loving, soft, and gentle, while other times we want to be fucked hard and long.

★ Obtain a 6-foot (1.8 m) rope.

★ Ahead of time, agree on a safety word, such as "potato chip," that signifies an end to all activity. This agreement will allow you to be creative and spontaneous while being respectful and safe. Do not rely on words such as "stop," because sometimes people confuse it with "don't stop" (as in "keep going").

THE LEAD-IN

Approach her with the intention to calm and alchemize. By design, you have a calming, masculine presence. The next time she is being bitchy for no reason, declare, "that's enough," carry her up the stairs, and playfully throw her on the bed.

THE FOREPLAY

① Grab her face with both hands and kiss her with gusto in the middle of her bitching session. Anger is just energy. Let it transform into lusty energy—the sexy kind.

② Flirtatiously pull down her pants and spank her bare ass. The vibrations from a spank on the behind give a nice hello to the entire clitoral network.

③ Bury your face in her crotch and moan and groan with energetic zest, sending tingles up her spine.

④ Press your gums against her commissure. Using a flat, relaxed tongue, move clockwise around the clitoris, licking with passion, and let her erotic desire surface.

⑤ Take off your pants in a feverish hurry. Take off her clothes with the same gusto. Read her energy. Listen for the safety word.

|||||||||||||||||||||||||||||||||||||||||||||||||||||||||||||||||||||||||||||||||||||||||||||||||||

SEX FACT

According to Askmen.com, force fantasy ranked third for top female fantasies.

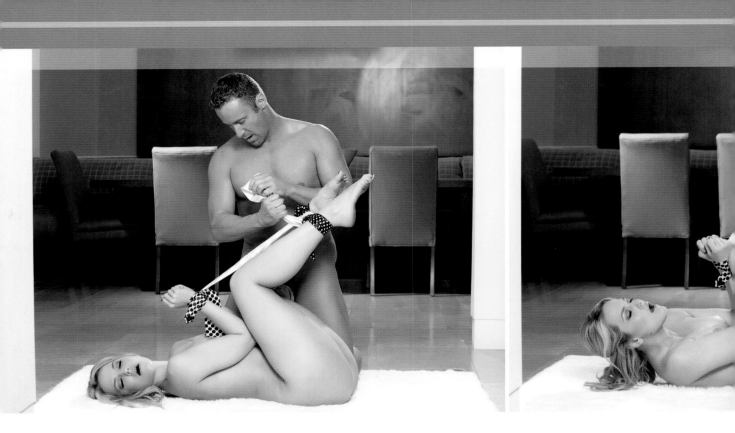

⭐ *The Main Act*

1 Lift her arms over her head and tie them together and hold them down. This is a move that is suggestive of you taking control.

2 With one hand holding down the rope and her chest wide open, scoot your body down and suck firmly on her breast. Command her to spread her legs as you open them suggestively with your hand.

3 Pump your cock inside directly with more speed and with a little force. She can moan and scream indecencies all she wants. When she does, give her a passionate kiss.

4 Does your wild one need to be tied up? If so, have her lie on her back and tie her ankles and hands together in a reverse hog tie. Start by bringing her hands in front of her (instead of behind) and tying them together using a soft sash, tie, or scarf. Then tie her feet together and join them to her hands, leaving her backside exposed. Get on your knees and penetrate. Reach up and grab her tied limbs with one hand and move them to the side. Experiment with different angles as you lower her arms and legs to each side. (See above.)

5 The elevation of the hog tie with her legs lifted will let you penetrate her deeply and ultimately hit her cervix zone. Penetrate slowly, because not all women enjoy cervix stimulation. Shallower thrusts will access her G-spot, another delightful zone you don't want to miss.

6 Alchemize the energy as you fuck, bitch, moan and groan yourselves back to normalcy.

7 Store the rope nearby. The next time you argue over something silly, lay the rope out for her to find and add a note with a heart on it.

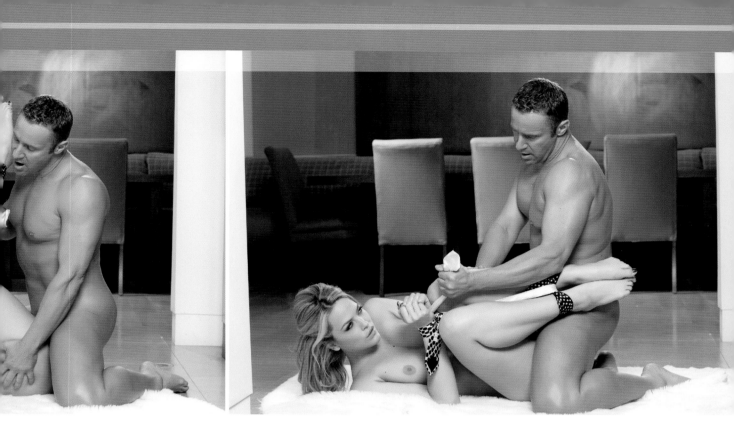

♀ WHY IT WORKS FOR HER

★ This position stimulates her G-spot and posterior fornix, both of which are along the same path of the vagina. The G-spot is about 2 inches (5 cm) inside the vagina and closer to the front of the body; the posterior fornix of the cervix is about 4 inches (10 cm) deep.

★ Many women were taught not to express or even feel anger—only more acceptable emotions, such as joy. Accepting her bitch once in a while is accepting all of her.

♂ WHY IT WORKS FOR HIM

★ Notice the quality of your erection when you give orders. Men usually report that being directive helps achieve and maintain an erection.

★ Deep thrusts give nice sensations to the head of your cock and full coverage to your shaft, and with vigorous pumping offers a nice balls massage.

RELATED MOVES

★ If you can't carry her to the bed, fuck the bitchiness out of her on the couch, a chair, or a table, or even standing in the kitchen!

||||||||||||||||||||||||||||||||||||||||||||||||||||||||||||||||||||||||||||||||||||||||||||||||||||||

THE SEXPERT SAYS

Many people find that when they are experiencing an intense emotion with their partner, their reaction is to shut down, blame, accuse, or withhold. Before you know it, the problem becomes bigger, both of you are exhausted, hard-ons and turn-ons are lost, and no one feels like having sex. Learn to let go and alchemize.

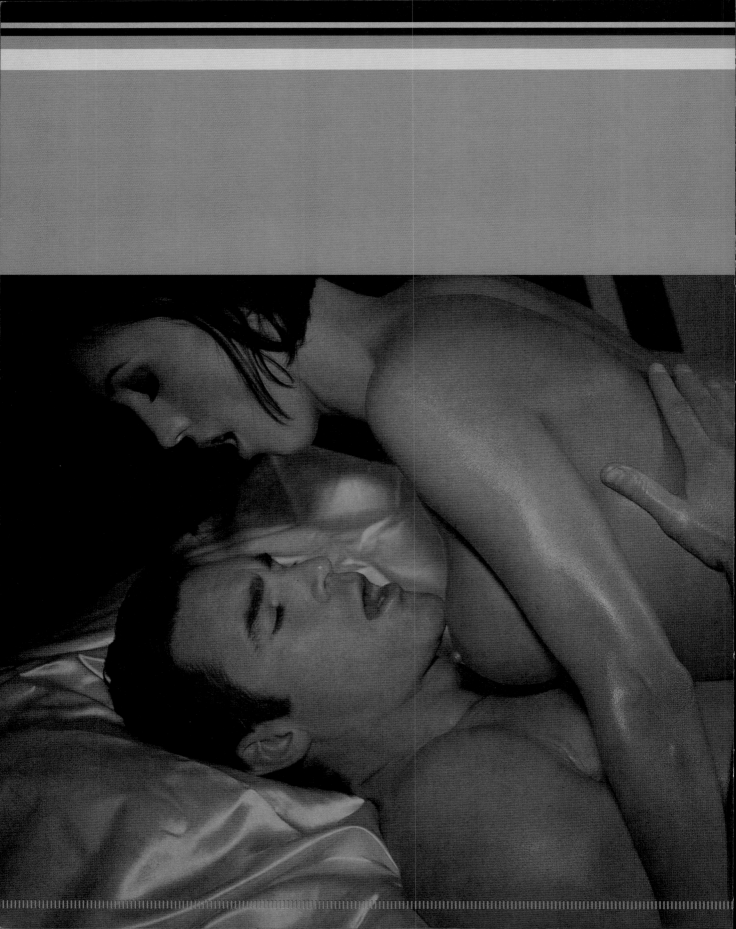

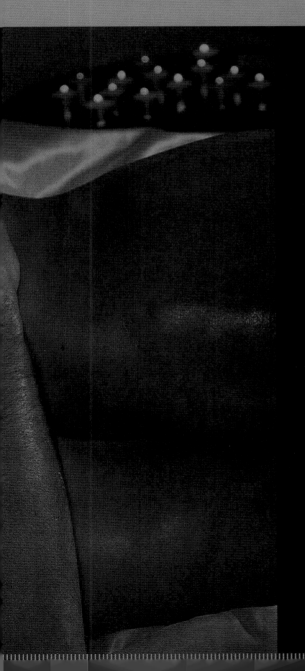

She's On Top

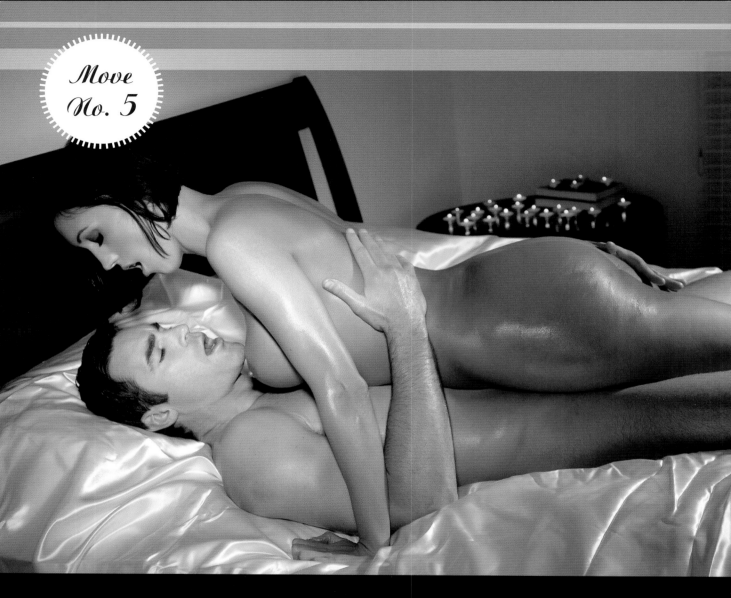

 # EASY GLIDER

Easy Glider is a sensational full-on body experience that you will remember and love for the full contact slip and glide that simultaneously massages both bodies. This scenario is perfect for nights when you both need a massage and can't decide whether to give or receive first.

The Move: Easy Glider

THE PREPARATIONS

★ Put baby oil by the bed or wherever you anticipate having sex.

★ Lay down a comforter, sheet, or towels you don't care about getting dirty.

★ Light some candles, put on some relaxing music, pour her a glass of wine, and lay out her robe. Get undressed and put on your robe.

THE LEAD-IN

When she walks in the door from the hustle and bustle, she will hear the music and see flickering candles and a note placed next to a robe that reads, "Get undressed and meet me in the bedroom."

THE FOREPLAY

1. There you both are, standing in your fluffy robes, only you are holding a bottle of baby oil. Motion for her to come over to you and open up her robe, then open your own. Take her hands and apply some baby oil and then place her oiled hands on your shoulders. She will get the hint.

2. After oiling up her hands, say, "Show me how you like it." We massage the way we like to receive massage, so now is your chance to put that theory to the test. When it's your turn to show how you like it, apply oil all over her body with long glorious strokes, especially the front. Spend extra time on erogenous spots: give wide cross strokes to her breasts and knead her butt.

3. Once you have lubed up her front side, lie down on your back and position her on top. Simultaneously give each other oral sex; ask her to use the same philosophy to show you how she likes to be licked.

||||||||||||||||||||||||||||||||||||||||||||||||||||||||||||||||||||||||||||||||||||||||||||||||||||||||

SEX FACT

Contrary to popular belief, the skin (not your penis) is the largest organ of the human body.

★ The Main Act

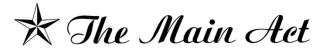

1 Once you are both fully aroused, lie down on the play sheets flat on your back with your legs fully extended.

2 Have her lie on top with her legs closed and also fully extended, allowing for a tight and full contact, skin-to-skin experience. Have her arms hold her upper body as she glides her body slowly over you and onto your slippery cock. Wow!

3 Tell her to put her hands by her sides in a push-up position and stiffen her body so she is moving all at once. Take hold of her hips and slowly glide her off your cock (all the way out of her vagina) and then all the way deep inside again and again. Did I say slowly?

4 She will feel the rub between her labia and the stimulation on her clit. You will feel the all-over body sensations, but notice the tightness of her vagina, the rubbing on your balls, and the sensation on the head of your penis each time you enter her closed labia.

5 Press her butt into you and hold it there. Notice the all-over body sensations and the sound of your heartbeats as you slip and glide. Mmmm. Hold on to her rear and maneuver her back and forth so she can enjoy intercourse and a clit massage.

6 Ready for a change of position? Tell her to lift her chest and press her pelvis down while she continues to thrust on your cock. This will provide shorter thrusts but deeper penetration and even more pressure on the clitoris. Look into her eyes. Rub a finger over her nipples.

7 Few things are sexier than hearing your lover's soft, sultry voice talking dirty. It's so sexy hot, it's enough to take her over the top. Using moans and groans, let her hear how it feels and why you love to fuck her.

8 Slow and steady are key to feeling this all-over body sensation, and the steadiness will help you and her find the rhythm for orgasm. It's quite possible that you will both climax together.

RELATED MOVES

★ For extra tightness, ask her to contract her PC muscle or grip your cock, particularly on the glide out.

★ Position yourself on top. Have her hold her feet out so you can use them as a footboard to slide up and down her body. On your way up, be sure to extend the glide so your pubic bone rubs on her clit.

♀ WHY IT WORKS FOR HER

★ The slipping and sliding full-body sensation, especially with her legs closed, lets her feel the glide on her outer labia, an often ignored but very sensitive spot. Also, this position provides a delicious combination of vaginal and clitoral massage.

♂ WHY IT WORKS FOR HIM

★ This position tickles a really nice spot on the head of your penis and massages the balls.

★ The teamwork required in this position will make it easy to establish a rhythm and possibly allow you to climax together.

||||||||||||||||||||||||||||||||||||||||||||||||||||||||||||||||||||||||||||||||||||||||||||||||||||||||||||||||||||||||

THE SEXPERT SAYS

Use your bedroom voice, talk dirty, or at least make moans and groans of enjoyment during sex so she knows what to repeat and continue doing. This is not only over-the-top hot, but also the immediate feedback will prove to be incredibly valuable for future sessions.

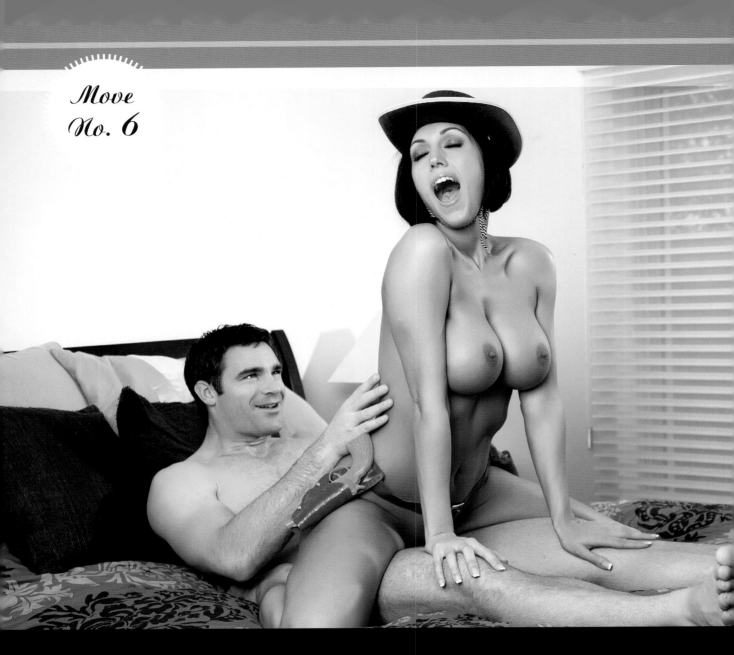

BUCKING BRONCO

This is one of the ultimate control moves for a woman on top. With her on top, use your strong arms to move her hips to and fro, and round and round, as you coach her to ride your cock, giving her the most bang for her buck. She will appreciate your involvement and rootin' tootin' cheers. Learn the tips and tricks that will make you her favorite bronco to buck.

The Move: Bucking Bronco

THE PREPARATIONS

★ Does she like country music? If so, make two CDs—one for you to play when she walks in the door and another to give her as part of the invitation.

★ If she has a key, post a note on the door that reads, "Please knock before entering." (You don't want her to ruin the surprise!)

★ Order take-out barbecue ribs (or faux ribs) and other Southern fixins and have it ready by the time she gets home, along with a box of hand wipes.

★ Lay a tarp down on the floor and take the food out of the box.

★ Time to get dressed. Cut out the back pockets from an old pair of tight jeans. Skip the underwear, slip on your homemade chaps, remove your shirt, and top it off with a cowboy hat.

★ Turn on the heat or light a fire if it's winter. Crank the music and be ready to answer the door. She is going to laugh her ass off with those chaps.

THE LEAD-IN

Early in the week, hand her your country CD in a jewel case and enclose a note that reads: "To my favorite cowgirl: Join me for a hootenanny at _____ (your place) on _____ (date and time)."

THE FOREPLAY

① Take her hand and walk over to the tarp. Turn to face her, grab her hand, and put it on your bare ass. Take off your hat and put it on her head. Take off the rest of your clothes until you are standing butt naked and give her an old-fashioned kiss.

② Grab a bone, smear the sauce on wherever you want to be licked, and ask her to give it a taste. Tell her that if she wants to stand in the naked zone, she must get naked, too.

③ Invite her to sit on the tarp and pass her the box of hand wipes for clean eating as you serve her.

④ Lick your fingers, and lick each other. The rule is if sauce falls on the body during the feeding it has to be licked up. Look out; sauce can get in the darnedest places. I dare you to get lost in the mess. But wherever the hootenanny takes you, have it end with you lying on your back and her sitting on your face.

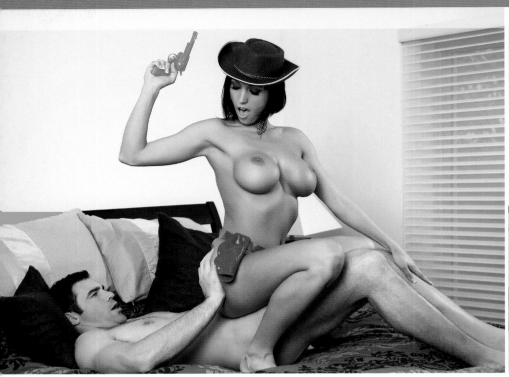
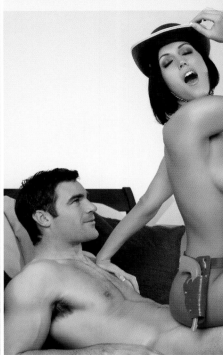

⭐ The Main Act

1 Still lying on your back, have her scoot down so she is on top and crouching over your body with her knees bent. In this position, her vagina is wide open for deep penetration and she can rub her breasts and clit on you as she desires.

2 Spread her ass cheeks open to tease her sphincter or slap her ass.

3 Roar and cheer as she rides your wild cock. Move your pelvis up and down, really bucking her.

4 Change the position a little. Sit up a bit so you are reclining on your elbows or are propped on a pillow. From this position, you can bring yourself in close to squeeze her breasts together and move your tongue back and forth between her nipples. She can also push against your chest for resistance and to find deeper penetration. Either one of you can stimulate her clit with your fingers.

5 For ultra-deep and controlled penetration, but no clitoral stimulation, guide her feet directly under her for a froglike position. Place your hands on her hips and help lift and lower her pussy onto your cock.

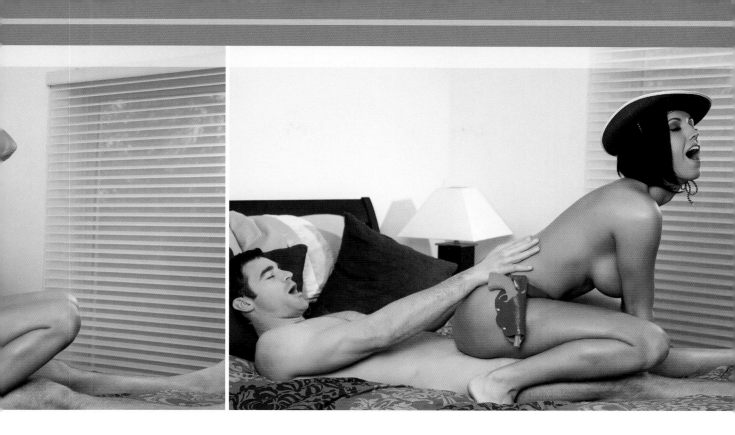

6 When you are both ready for a pause, maybe from fatigue or because you don't want to climax just yet, have her sit straight up with her hands behind her. Stimulate her breasts while she squeezes her PC muscle and milks your penis. I find that sexual intercourse is one of the best times to get your Kegel reps in because you have instant feedback. Do your PC exercises, too. Ask her to reach back and play with your testicles.

7 When you're ready, direct her to the reverse cowgirl position. Reverse cowgirl is the traditional woman-on-top position, but instead of being positioned face-to-face, you are looking at her back and she is facing your toes. (See above.)

8 Get into this position slowly and carefully by asking her to contract her PC muscle while your cock is deep inside her. You will need to guide her by lifting up one of her legs, gently moving it in the direction you want her to go, and asking her to turn around slowly. She may not be familiar with this position and the range of motion of your penis. Have her get into the position without you pulling out. It's sort of like a slow sit and spin. She can maintain her balance by placing her hands in front of her. She will get to feel oh so nice pressure and sensations in different spots in the vagina.

9 Put your hands on her shoulders and encourage her to lean back, or for gyration, hold on to her hips and move her back and forth. Try making circles by holding her waist and guiding her with your hands.

10 From the reverse cowgirl, do a slight turn so she is at seven o'clock or four o'clock (depending on which way she turns); her shoulder should be facing you and she should be straddling your leg, which allows her to rub it on her clit. This position will rub your cock in all the right ways, while having the familiar stroke on her clit.

11 Slowly turn her sidesaddle or to nine o'clock or three o'clock, so her heels are touching your ass cheek. In this position, she can have her knees bent for deeper penetration or have her legs out in front of her for more tightness. For extra tightness have her close her legs.

12 Now, repeat the process and take this position 360 degrees around the cock, counterclockwise and to orgasm.

RELATED MOVES

★ Once she's on top of you, in the upright position, have her lean back on her elbows. At this point she can push off her elbows for a deeper thrust and you can stimulate her wide-open clitoris.

★ From the reverse cowgirl, have her lean back onto you, her back against your chest, with her knees slightly bent; she may need to guide her pelvis down onto your cock. Grab her breasts from behind and play with her nipples or move your hand down to fondle her clit.

SEX FACT

According to sex researcher Sandra Leiblum, Ph.D., people who do the same thing in bed are the ones who report that sex is boring. Sometimes all we need is to switch it up a little to spice up our sex lives.

♀ WHY IT WORKS FOR HER

★ Being on top offers excellent G-spot stimulation and complete control, which means increased satisfaction and possibly multiple orgasms. She can have more or less clitoral stimulation by leaning forward and rubbing on your pubic bone. She can monitor the depth and pace of penetration by how she moves her hips.

♂ WHY IT WORKS FOR HIM

★ You are going to love the view of her ass from this position and seeing what your girl does when you give her the reins.

★ Also, the women-on-top position gives you better control because the blood and energy are drawn away from your penis.

||||||||||||||||||||||||||||||||||||||||||||||||||||||||||||||||||||||||||||||||||||||||||||||||||||||||||||||||||||||||||||

THE SEXPERT SAYS

Another reason this position offers better control is because you can relax your pelvic muscles. Muscle tension is a normal part of the orgasmic phase of the sexual response cycle. So, if you want to lengthen the phase or delay orgasm, it makes sense to reduce muscle tension.

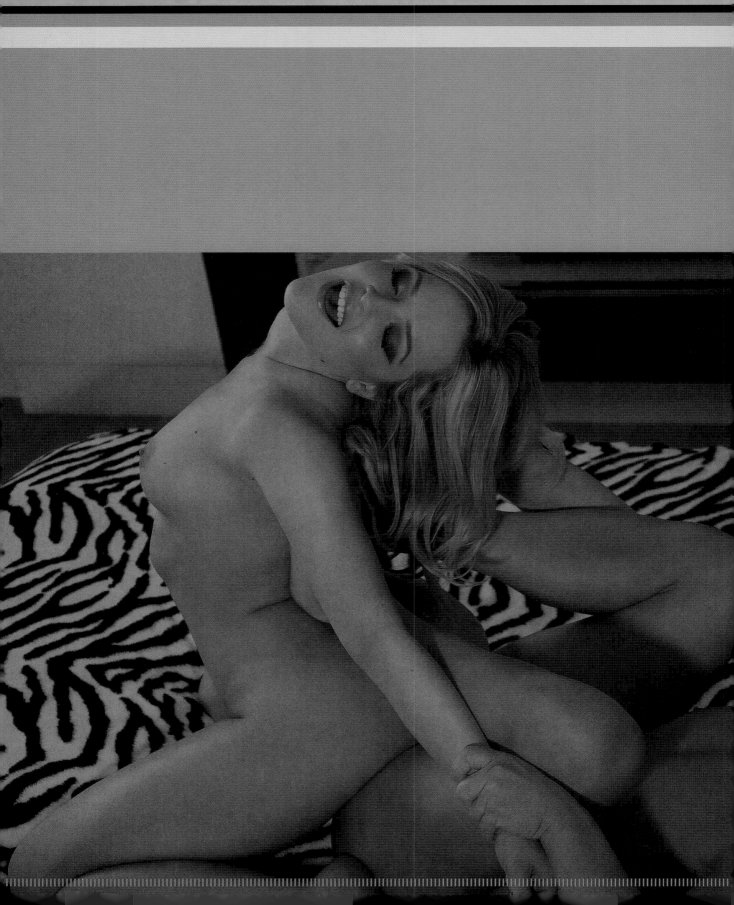

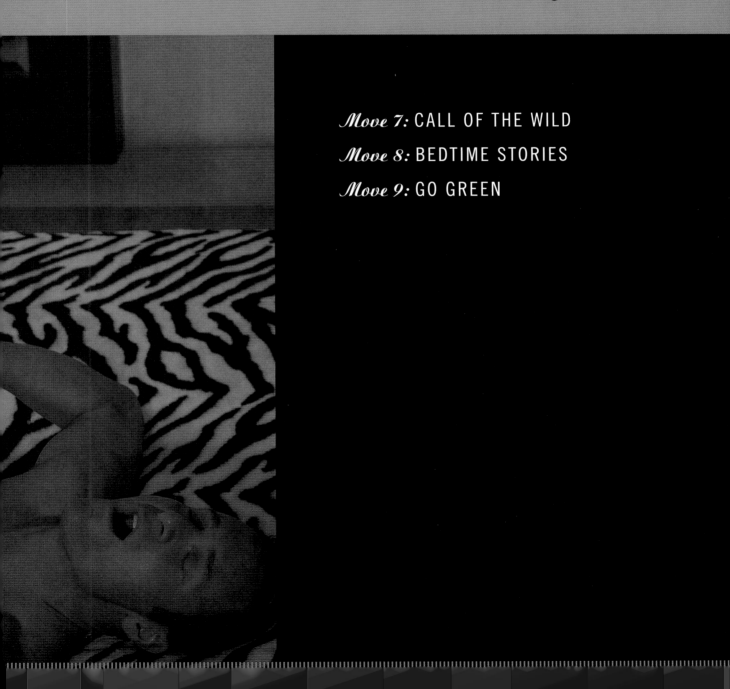

Rear Entry

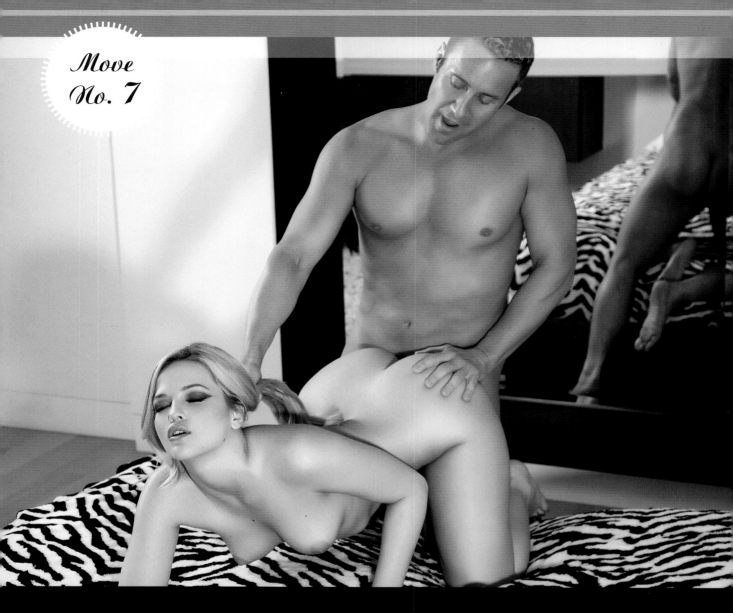

 # CALL OF THE WILD

Howl and growl, grunt and moan as you do it wild animal style. Grab her hair and take her on a wild safari where she can encounter her carnal side and set it free. Discover the rear-entry variations that the best of the beasts know to get her growling with delight.

Most women have a secret desire to be wildly ravished by their partner and let go totally

The Move: Call of the Wild

THE PREPARATIONS

★ Rent or buy a movie that depicts wild animals mating. Watch it before showing it to her so you can cue it to the best scenes.

★ Clean the house so she can relax into the fantasy. She doesn't really want to make love in a dirty house, even though wild animals wouldn't care.

★ Do you ever want to go wild, animalistic, and instinctive on your girl? Guess what? She probably wants that, too, once in a while. Ask her. Give yourselves permission to let go and totally ravish each other. You may have to be the one to put yourself out there and be a little silly at first, but trust me: it's all worth it.

THE LEAD-IN

Cue up the movie and sit down on the couch in your robe. When she sits down to join you press play on your DVD and take off your robe to let your wild animal roam—arrrgggghhh!

When you are both turned on, give her a sample of your best animal mating call. Growl in her ear and pant on her neck.

THE FOREPLAY

① Curl up next to her and growl. Nuzzle your snout in her neck and give her a love bite. Move that snout to her crotch. Bite on her pants, claw her shirt, and give a roar to imply that she remove them or risk having her favorite panties eaten in the struggle.

② Although you don't want to rip or tear her clothes, remove any clothing in a rough kind of way.

③ Thrust your pelvis against her, making wild animal sounds. Grab her by the hair (more symbolism, less pain) and take her down to the floor on all fours.

④ Get behind her on the ground and do what all animals do when they see another animal's rear: smell her. While you are there, lick her rear.

⑤ From here, you can take the lead of the wild beasts on the video, or go on your own Kama Sutra animal safari. Most of the positions in the Kama Sutra are named after animals and nature, mirroring our relationship with the natural world.

||||||||||||||||||||||||||||||||||||||||||||||||||||||||||||||||||||||||||||||||||||||||

SEX FACT

Retro canino is Latin for "doggy style," or sex from behind.

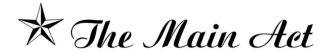

The Main Act

THE DOG

1 While she is on all fours, kneel behind her, hold her hair, grip her waist, and enter her from behind. Let out a sound that matches how it feels to penetrate her.

2 To feel her tight, have her close her legs and tighten her ass and PC muscle. To feel her loose, open her legs and tell her to bare down slightly or relax her PC muscle. To feel her deep, grab her shoulder or hips and pull her into you.

3 Pay attention to how she moves on the safari. Is she thrusting back toward you in a quicker motion? She wants it faster. Is she pushing back into you, wanting it deeper? Is she crawling away, wanting it shallower? Is she moving from side to side? She wants the wild cat position.

THE WILD CAT

1 Show her who the king of the jungle is. Have her lie on her stomach and penetrate her from behind. Have her bend her knees so her ankles are near your hands, then lift her ankles and rock slowly from side to side. (See near right.)

THE ELEPHANT

1 Have her lie down so that you can enter her from behind. She can leave her legs open for easier penetration, or tighten her thighs to firmly squeeze on your penis.

2 Time to turn it hot with the friskiest of them all, hot monkey love.

HOT MONKEY LOVE

1 Lie on your back and bend your knees toward your face. Have your lover sit on your thighs with her back to you; press your feet against her shoulders so she can use them as a backrest. Her arms should be pointing back toward you while you hold her wrists. (See far right.)

RELATED MOVES

★ It's true: wild animals go for their own pleasure, but there are many opportunities to stimulate her nipples and clit. Many animals masturbate, so you can also roar for her to stroke herself.

★ Instead of vaginal entry, an obvious related move would be anal entry. If you do go for anal entry, you might find that she will be more relaxed and get more pleasure if you give her an oral orgasm first.

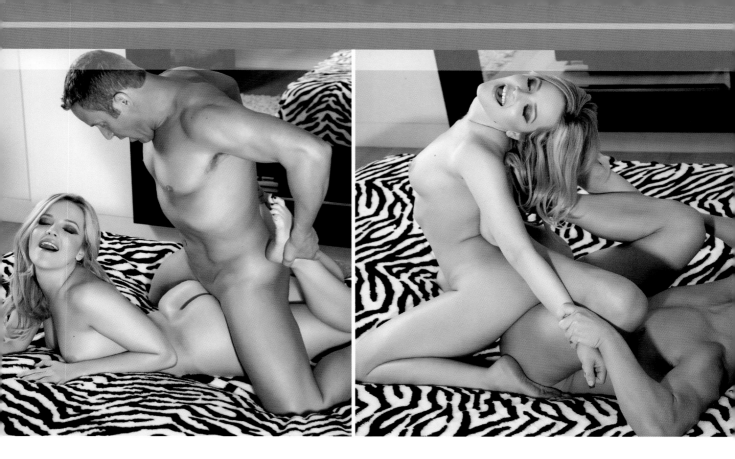

♀ WHY IT WORKS FOR HER

★ There is a lot of rear-entry variety here and opportunities to stimulate different places in her vagina. Following her lead and maneuvering the position of her legs will be the keys to that.

♂ WHY IT WORKS FOR HIM

★ You'll get great views of her rear and many mounting opportunities. Also, notice what the commanding, wild animal persona does for the quality of your erection.

||||||||||||||||||||||||||||||||||||||||||||||||||||||||||||||||||||||||||||||||||||||||||||||||||||||||||||||

THE SEXPERT SAYS

If you set the intention for lovemaking, that's what you will get, even if it is fast, howling, growling, romping, and a little wild. Commit to spending a block of time together each night making love or completely ravishing each other.

||||||||||||||||||||||||||||||||||||||||||||||||||||||||||||||||||||||||||||||||||||||||||||||||||||||||||||||

SEX FACT

The San Diego Zoo leads tours of mating animals on Valentine's Day. It sells out each year.

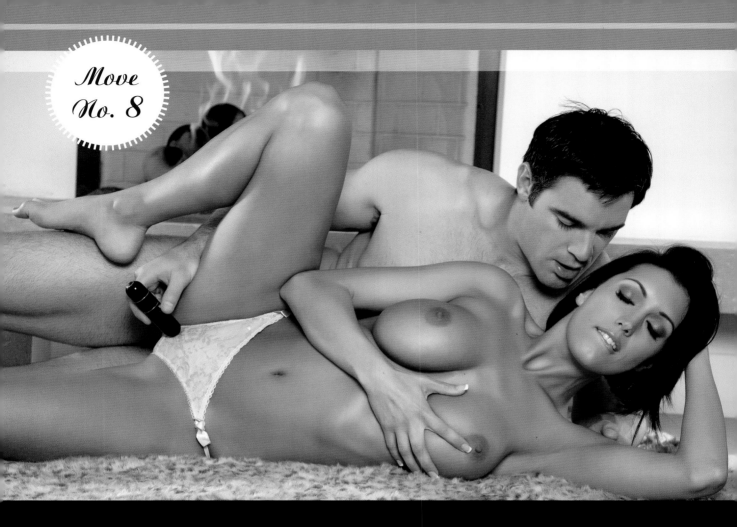

 # BEDTIME STORIES

Tuck her in with sweet dreams as you let her know who is in charge (at least for the moment) with this subtle but directive scenario that ignites her erotic mind and satisfies her physical needs. She is folded over with her knees to her chest as you mount her and read an erotic submission story.

Women love words. Hearing you whisper erotica in her ear while being wrapped in your arms of safety and filled with your cock is a hard combo to beat. You don't need to be a Casanova for this one. Simply choose your story and read. You have the room and freedom to try things you

The Move: Bedtime Stories

THE PREPARATIONS

★ Ideally, you would make up your own submission story. If you are looking for some good ideas or full-on stories, check out Rachel Kramer Bussel's erotica. Choose a few you like and mark the pages.

★ Gather some warming lube or a clitoral stimulating gel and a vibrating bullet and place them under your pillow.

★ Do a practice reading and get into character. It's interesting to note comfort levels. If being directive is difficult for you, practice making directive statements while holding the intention of love.

★ Knowing how your penis responds not only to your own touch but also to your thoughts and energy is important information and can be helpful when you want to achieve or maintain an erection. One thought can give a man an erection and one thought can take it away. What are those thoughts for you?

THE LEAD-IN

Instead of turning over for the night, turn it on. Pull out the book and pull up behind her for a nice spoon and tell her that you want to read her a bedtime story.

THE FOREPLAY

① Start off spooning her from behind so she is relaxed in the fetal position. Kiss her neck and ears as you relish in the nighttime reading with your sweetie.

② Begin to read your custom story. Randomly and playfully narrate your own lines in the story so you can apply the lube: "He gently caressed her begging breasts, her nipples perched like peaks of a mountain. He reached down and could feel the heat from her vivacious vulva as he pushed her panties aside to gently massage her and spread the wetness." Let the giggles come and go but don't stop—keep reading.

③ Reach around with one hand and gently pinch her labia together, moving your thumb and index finger together. This gives her a massage to her labia.

THE SEXPERT SAYS

We all experience moments when we would like for our lovers or ourselves to be more dominant or more submissive. This scenario helps us try on new roles.

Insert an index finger into her vagina for some natural lube and bring your finger up and around, circling the clitoris. Now repeat the same gentle pinch you did with the labia to the crura and base of the clitoris. When she shows increased signs of arousal, such as lubrication, increased breathing, and/or perspiration, begin running your index finger up and down the clitoral shaft with light pressure over the clitoral glans.

(4) Place a vibrating bullet inside her panties to hold or maintain clitoral stimulation.

★ The Main Act

1 With a gentle hand, guide her into position: her knees are to her chest and she is face down with her head on the pillow. (In yoga circles it would look similar to child's pose.) Drape yourself over her back, mounting her, and begin reading the sexy story.

2 You are following the intention of the main male character. Each time the main character asserts himself, do the same: stroke her hair and then give it a gentle pull. Kiss her neck and then give her a little bite. If he ties her up, put her arms above her head, kiss her neck, and suck her nipples.

3 Rub your cock up against her ass as if you are going to insert it into her anus, but don't. Reach in and rub her clitoris, using lube if necessary.

4 If he licks the damsel, you lick your damsel.

5 At the pinnacle of the story, when the man penetrates, you penetrate her with your cock. Lower your pelvis down for an increased range of motion and greater depth. Shallower pumps will access her G-spot because it is closer to the vaginal entrance, while deeper pumps will access her cervix, which is at the back wall of the vagina.

6 If you use the vibrating bullet, simply push the panties aside for insertion.

7 Spread her legs for a looser fit and close them for a tighter one.

8 Cue her in to what you want her to do: "She grips his cock by contracting her PC muscle and then she releases him by relaxing them."

9 Put the book down and ask her what comes next, letting her finish the erotic story with her own imagination as you tickle her clit and fantasize her to orgasm.

10 Wrap her in your arms and read the rest of the story throughout resolution as you kiss, hug, and snuggle her.

SEX FACT

Number of hours per day the TV is on in an average U.S. home: 6 hours, 47 minutes. (Who has time for sex?)

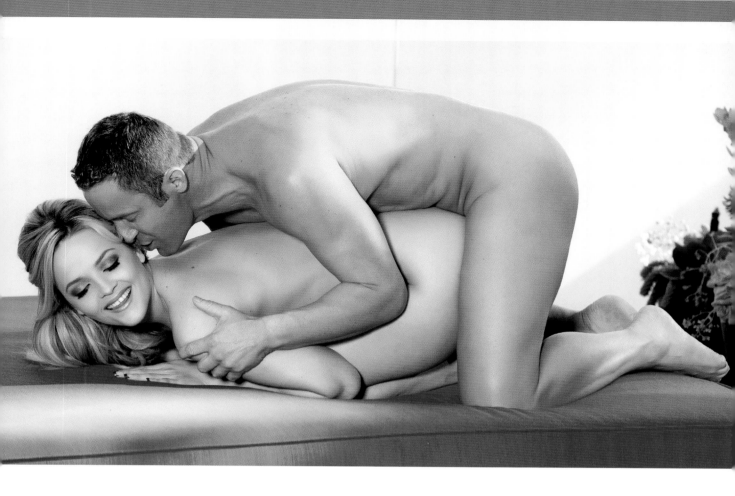

RELATED MOVES

★ Switch positions/roles and let her be dominant with a dildo or strap-on and lots of lube. You might get some ideas on how she likes to be managed.

★ Let her choose a story for you to read, or randomly open a page and seek adventure together.

★ You can also do anal entry instead of vaginal.

♀ WHY IT WORKS FOR HER

★ The rear-entry position is great for both G-spot and cervix stimulation.

★ This rear position is perfect for letting her mind wander with fantasy.

★ It's ultra hot to hear the voice of the hero of her choice reading erotica, blanketed by your body and filled with your cock.

♂ WHY IT WORKS FOR HIM

★ Your shaft feels "gripped" or massaged when she closes her legs or contracts her PC muscle.

★ You will learn the power of your words and the effect it has on her arousal.

★ You can expand your repertoire to be someone else for a change.

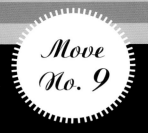

Move No. 9

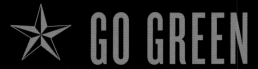

★ GO GREEN

Sprinkler sex is a refreshing solution on a hot day. And what brings back fond memories of playing in the grass? Sprinklers and wheelbarrow races. She has her hands on the grass, while you are standing and holding her legs like the handles of a wheelbarrow, penetrating her from the rear while the sprinkler showers her clitoris. Try different sprinklers and you might discover a fresh surprise on your own equipment.

Who says that you are too old to play in the sprinkler, and who says it's too hot for sex? Nonsense.

The Move: Go Green

THE PREPARATIONS

★ Set up the sprinklers in your backyard. You can use a toy sprinkler that simply attaches to a hose as long as it has a nice spray with lots of pressure. Buy several and choose your favorite.

★ Or, if you live in an apartment, or you want to spice up suburbia, notice when the nighttime sprinklers go on at your local playing field and take a drive to play in your bathing suit.

★ Some women masturbate with streams of water from a bathtub, detachable shower head, or hot tub. Does your girl like to play with water? Find out.

★ Turn on the sprinkler, turn off the lights, blend a piña colada, and put on some dance music.

||||||||||||||||||||||||||||||||||||||||||||||||||||||||||||||||||||||||||||||||||||||||||||||||||||||

SEX FACT

Rheononia is female masturbation using a stream of water.

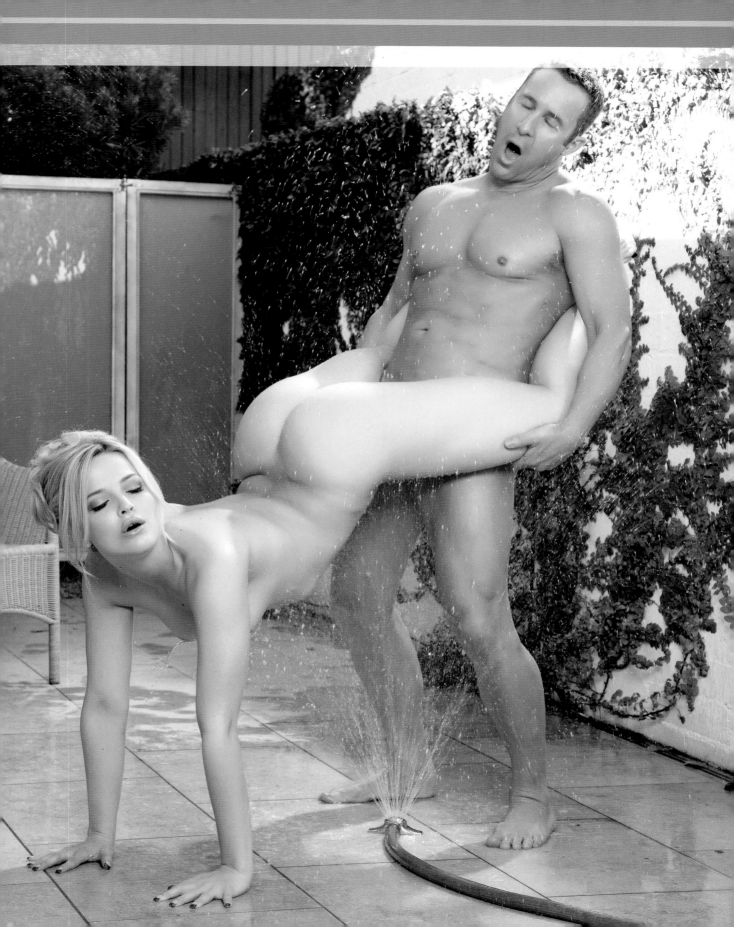

THE LEAD-IN

The next time it's too hot to sleep, don't turn to the air conditioner for relief; go for sprinkler sex.

Tell her to grab her bathing suit and meet you out in the backyard (or car, if you live in an apartment and will drive to a playing field) in 10 minutes for a surprise. No peeking.

THE FOREPLAY

1. The foreplay here is fun. Run, hop, jump, and skip through the sprinklers with the carefree abandonment you had as a kid.

2. If it is a directional sprinkler, hold hands and run under or jump over the sprinkler.

3. Shimmy and shake in the sprinkler to your favorite song.

4. Stop and hold her from behind, positioning her over the sprinkler while you give her a kiss on the neck so she knows you mean business.

5. If she is wearing a suit, push the bottoms aside and give her a nice genital massage with your fingers.

6. Sit her upright on her knees and directly over the sprinkler while you are standing in front of her. Stroke your penis and ask if she will give you a blow job.

7. Her turn. Position her on all fours and directly over the sprinkler, while you are on your knees licking her rear and reaching your arms forward to stimulate her nipples.

|||||||||||||||||||||||||||||||||||||||||||||||||||||||||||||||||||||||||||||||||||||||||||||||||||||||||||||

THE SEXPERT SAYS

Adults love surprises as much as children do. Don't limit them to birthdays and holidays. Playing with water takes you back to your childhood, giving you a sense of fun and freedom to be silly and let your guard down. My wish is that you do moves like this one and feel inspired to experiment and create your own sexual masterpieces.

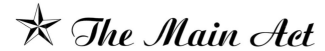# ★ *The Main Act*

1 Sit up and lean on her as you enter her from the rear. For more intense sprinkler stimulation on her clit, have her spread her knees and lower herself so she hovers over the sprinkler while you penetrate her from behind.

2 Spend most of your time here, because the wheelbarrow position requires strength from you and her, so she may not be able to sustain the inverted position for very long.

3 To move into the wheelbarrow stance, stand up from the kneeling position, and raise her waist so she is in an inverted "V." (In yoga circles this would look like downward dog.) Enjoy this position for a while.

4 When the time is right, ask her to lift and bend one of her legs, so her legs look like those of a flamingo standing on one leg. Grab that leg and play here for a while; open it for a looser fit and close it for a tighter one. See what happens if she crosses her bent knee in front of her.

5 When you are ready for the wheelbarrow, tell her to kick her standing leg up for you to grab. You're now holding both her legs while she balances her weight on her arms. Choke up on her legs so your hands are above her knees and closer to her waist.

6 Move your hands in closer and grab her waist, pulling her into you so you both splish and splash to orgasm.

7 Wrap her in a dry towel and hold her in your arms throughout resolution.

RELATED MOVES

★ Instead of resting her weight on her hands, she can rest her weight on her elbows.

♀ WHY IT WORKS FOR HER

★ Stimulation with water is delightful, and for some women it is their chosen masturbation style. Depending on the type of spray, the entire exterior of her vulva gets a water massage. Pair this with the deep insertion of your penis in the wheelbarrow position and you have a refreshing combo.

♂ WHY IT WORKS FOR HIM

★ Your hands can't be everywhere, but in this scenario her clit will be taken care of by the spray of the water while you enter from the rear and get ultra-hot sensations with her leg movements changing up the grip on your penis.

★ Experience a refreshing spray on your balls, perineum, and ass. Bidet anyone?

★ The standing positions and physical exertion require you to contract your muscles, which can help intensify both of your orgasms.

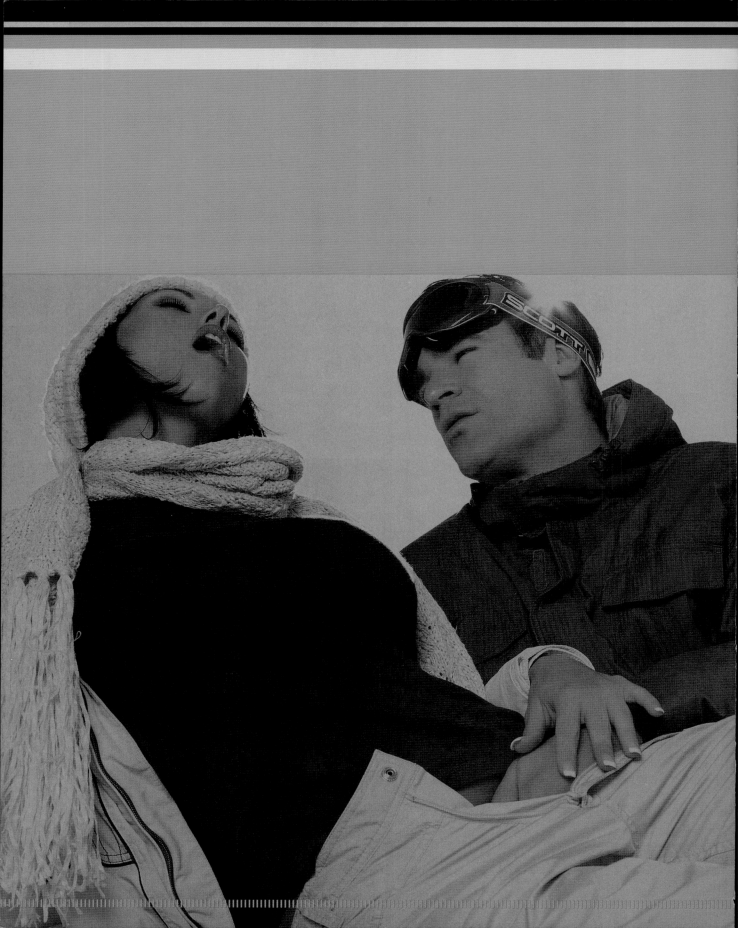

Sitting & Kneeling

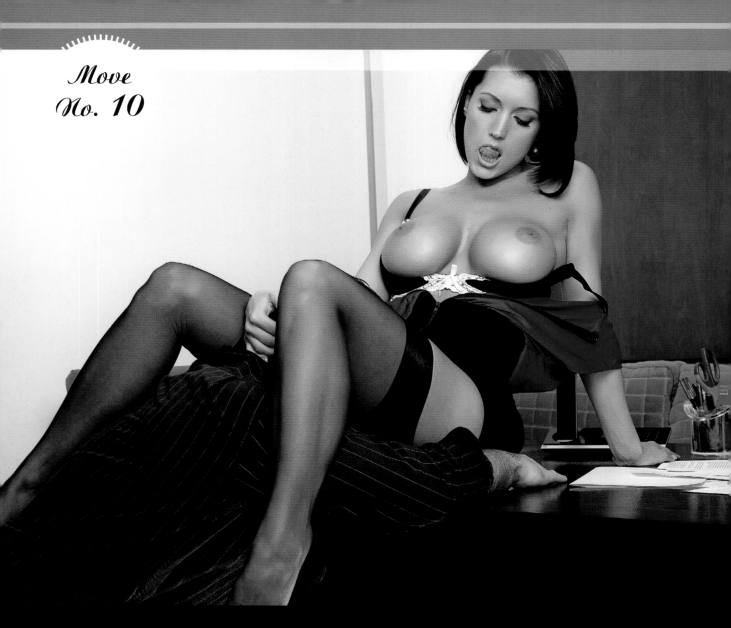

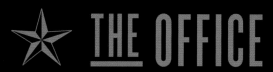

⭐ THE OFFICE

The office chairs with wheels come with great adjustments that allow for maximum leverage, increased depth of penetration, and better performance as you move her toward and away from you. This scenario is perfect for the girl who works late at the office or brings any kind of work

The Move: The Office

THE PREPARATIONS

★ Ask questions about her workplace, or go there to take her out to lunch and scope it out. Does anyone work late or on the weekends?

THE LEAD-IN

Pick out some beautiful flowers and set up a delivery at her office. If desired, include the following text: "Research shows that physical activity during the workday increases productivity, concentration, and cognitive skills; boosts performance; and allows for more tolerance and forgiveness. I am coming by at _____ (weekend or after hours) for your mandatory work break."

Alternatively, have lunch delivered to her home or work office at about 11 a.m. Follow it up with a text including the language above.

This will give her a chance to get excited and work double time so she can have an extended work break with you.

THE FOREPLAY

① She knows why you are there, so get to business. When she opens the office door, walk in and close the door behind you, declaring that you are there for the mandatory work break. Break time starts immediately as you kiss and suck on her neck. Open her blouse and kiss across her shoulder as you run your fingers down along the curve of her breasts and over her stomach.

② Get on your knees on the floor and slowly remove her shoes, skirt, and stockings one by one. Lick and fondle her legs, grab her ass, and dart your tongue over her clit as you erotically remove her clothes.

③ Once she's undressed from the waist down, have her lean against the desk, and pull her legs up to your shoulders. Move your nose around her clit, then use your tongue and apply consistent motion that feels good without sending her into orgasmic contractions just yet.

④ Keep licking her, darting your tongue in and out for clitoral stimulation, and alternate with kissing her vulva and inner thighs and massaging her ass.

‖‖

SEX FACT

Research shows that physical activity during the workday increases productivity, concentration, and cognitive skills; boosts performance; and allows for more tolerance and forgiveness. (Double the benefits when the physical activity is sexual in nature!)

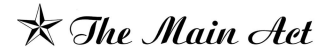 The Main Act

1 Support her desk chair to keep it from falling back. If it has wheels, lock them.

2 Sit in the chair and have her sit on your lap, straddling and facing you for your office merger. Her arms can be on your shoulders or the back of the chair as she grinds and rides you. Hold her at the waist to aid her up and down. If they fit, her legs are going to be between the chair arms and the seat. (See near right.)

3 Go for comfort. If her legs don't fit between the arms of the chair, have her sit on your lap, facing away from you and riding reverse cowgirl using the desk for support. With her positioned on top and her feet on the ground, she has control over the depth and direction of the merger.

4 Switch positions and angles by standing her up; she should have one leg on the chair and one leg on the ground and hold on to the back of the chair as you insert from behind and look at her assets. (See far right.)

5 Now have her put her other leg down while she is bent over the chair and show her entire portfolio. For even deeper penetration, you stand and take her from behind.

6 Place the chair up against the desk so it doesn't tip. Have her kneel on both knees on the chair with her hands holding on to the chair back. You hold her down as you climb on and insert from the rear, showing her who the boss is.

7 Have her sit on the desk while you stand, then bring her to orgasm as you pull her onto your penis. Lean forward to stroke her breasts with your fingertips or tickle her nipples with your chest. Have her recline with her knees to your chest for deeper penetration or rotate her bent knees from side to side for different sensations in the vulva.

RELATED MOVES

★ Add some role-play to your scenario: you play the seductive boss and she is the employee whom you are requiring to take a break, or she is the demanding boss and you are the assistant who needs to keep your job by satisfying her every whim, or some other male/female work-related scenario that turns you on.

★ If the desk is at least one foot lower than your penis, lay her flat on her back with her feet on your shoulders, then raise and lower her on your cock.

WHY IT WORKS FOR HER

♀ ★ She will think twice about working on a Saturday or maybe work more, considering the rewards.

★ Her being on top in the chair allows her to control the depth of the position and direction of the work break.

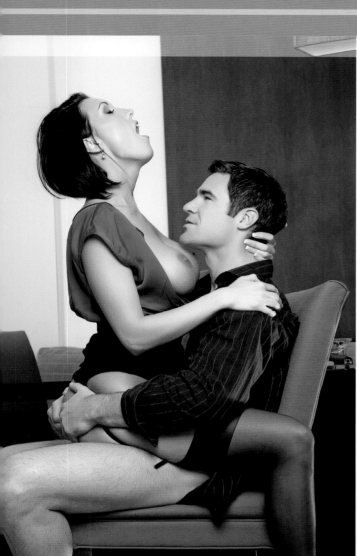
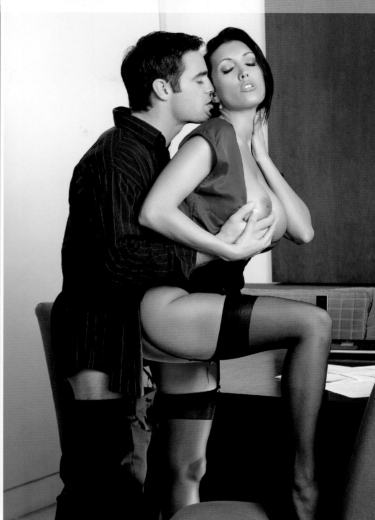

♂ WHY IT WORKS FOR HIM

★ The depth and penetration that office chairs offer is undeniable for you. With all the variety and possible combinations, you are sure to find an angle you can do every time she works overtime.

★ Having sex with your partner in the office totally shifts the energy of the office. It's like office feng shui without having to move the furniture.

|||||||||||||||||||||||||||||||||||||||||||||||||||||||||||||||||||||||||||||||||||||||||||||||||||||||

THE SEXPERT SAYS

It's so easy to get into a grind and think that work *is* our life. There is so much more to the art of living than just working and our routines. This scene helps give her a break and hopefully a new perspective.

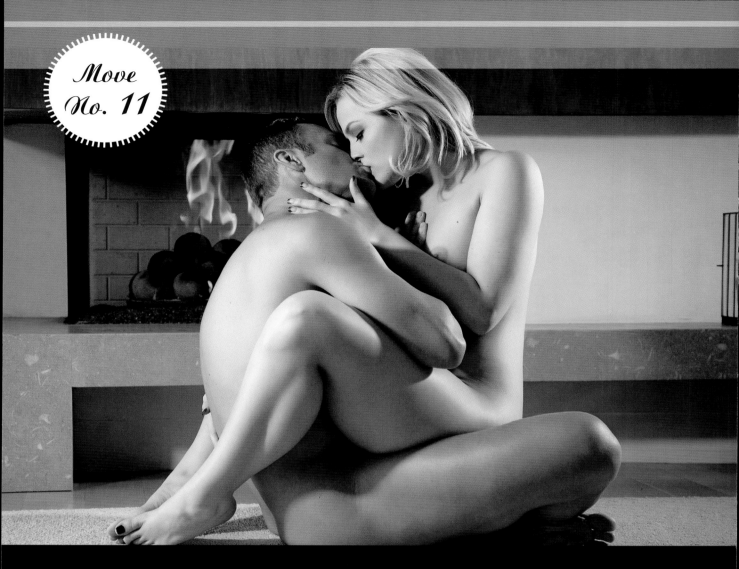

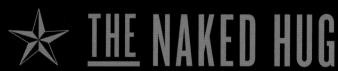

THE NAKED HUG

Do you ever ask your girl what is wrong, only to get the answer "nothing"? You know something is up and so does she, but she is looking for that safe space to surrender and open her heart with you, or maybe she just wants a hug. Lucky for you, you do not need to say anything except "everything is going to be okay" and put her in a position of intimacy, safety, and surrender.

You sit cross-legged and she sits on top, facing you, with her legs wrapped around you. She will love the simple touch that moves energy through the body, making for a more intense and lasting orgasm.

The Move: The Naked Hug

THE PREPARATIONS

★ Light candles around the room. For increased light, place them in front of a mirror.

★ Turn on the heater if it is cool. Gather some small sitting pillows and arrange them in the middle of the room.

★ Play relaxing yoga or meditation music. All of these things will help anchor her for calm and relaxation.

THE LEAD-IN

When you notice that your presence, caring, and nurturing are needed and she doesn't want to part from your embrace, give her the healing powers of skin-to-skin contact and suggest that you both remove your clothes for a naked hug.

THE FOREPLAY

① Connect with an embrace as soon as skin-to-skin contact becomes available. Offer to sit down on the pillows to be more comfortable for your embrace.

② Rest her head on your chest and rub your fingers through her hair. Gently rock her back and forth. Hold her face in your hands and kiss her forehead, her eyes, her lips, and her neck.

③ Give long strokes up and down her back. Kiss her shoulders and her breasts.

||||||||||||||||||||||||||||||||||||||||||||||||||||||||||||||||||||||||||||||||||||||||||||||||||||||||||||||||||||||||||||||||||||||||

SEX FACT

When we touch, our brain releases oxytocin, also known as the cuddle hormone, which decreases stress and increases our sexual responsiveness. Hormones create positive feedback loops, so the more you have, the more you want. The lesson is to touch regardless of whether you are feeling sexual or not.

★ The Main Act

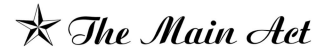

1. Sit with your legs crossed on the floor or on another firm surface. You can use a seat cushion or firm pillow under her bum if it is more comfortable.

2. Have her sit on your lap, facing you, with her legs wrapped around you. Adjust the wrap of her legs. Wrapping them too tightly will pull her in really close, bringing her body weight with her.

3. Have each of you place your right hand behind the other's neck and your left hand on the other's tailbone. You are in the perfect position for intimacy. Make eye contact, listen for each other's heartbeat, and kiss her with an open mouth while one of you breathes in and the other breathes out. This is very soothing and doable. You can also place a hand on each other's heart.

4. For instant intimacy, match your breathing to hers and deepen your breaths.

5. Insert your penis into her vagina. Do Kegels (squeeze and release your PC muscle) as you rock the hips together slowly back and forth. Rub your hand up and down each other's back.

6. Maintain eye contact as you kiss and build the rocking pace to orgasm. Hold the naked hug throughout resolution and wait for her to break the embrace.

THE SEXPERT SAYS

I often suggest that clients set aside time each day for sex. It doesn't have to be sexual intercourse and it doesn't have to be to orgasm. You simply want to create the time and space to connect so that sex can happen. This position is great because it includes intimacy and touching, and it can be done with a semierect penis.

RELATED MOVES

★ You can sit with your legs extended in front of you and her legs wrapped around you.

★ Alternatively, bend your knees and sit on your ankles with the soles of your feet facing up. She can sit in your lap, facing you, but have her bend her legs and place her ankles at your knees. This allows for more skin-to-skin contact but less depth. She can rub her breasts on your chest and her clit on your pelvis. It may also be more comfortable.

★ For further variation, sit on your rears, facing each other with hands behind your backs for balance. Have her rest her ankles on your shoulders. This position offers one of the deepest types of penetration, aiming the head of the penis at the posterior fornix.

♀ WHY IT WORKS FOR HER

★ This position (and the variations) can't be beaten for instant intimacy and connection. Your bodies are connected continuously, touching everywhere. This is also a good exercise when you want to experience more balance and shared power in your relationship.

♂ WHY IT WORKS FOR HIM

★ This position works well with a semierect penis or a hard one. Because it provides so much intimacy, which she craves, you can start from here and try variations for deeper or different penetration when your penis becomes more erect.

★ This position is very good for men who have a tendency to ejaculate early because it helps you slow down and be in the moment.

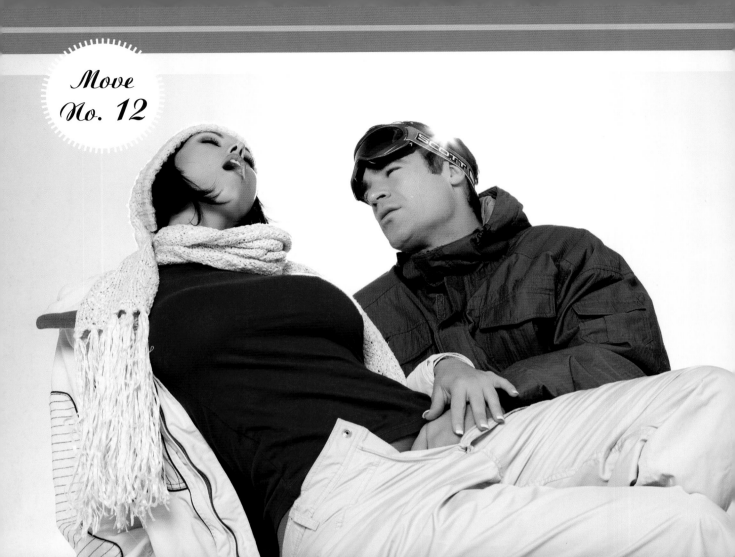

 # OH <u>MY</u> GONDOLA

Provide the perfect accompaniment to that great view on the gondola ride. She sits on your lap while you stroke her clitoris to orgasm. You have this angle down. Years of stroking your cock from the seated position will come in handy to give you added dexterity and confidence.

Every adventure is more fun with the idea of sex in the mix, especially cold-weather activities such as a bone-chilling gondola ride. Warm up the day and add a new perspective on

The Move: Oh My Gondola

THE PREPARATIONS

★ Pack a pocket rocket, hand warmer, and clitoral warming gel.

★ Find out how long the ski run takes. Don't make it your objective to give her an orgasm on the first lift ride. It will be more exciting to let the clitoral stimulating gel do its work while she heads down the slopes, then give her a little taste on each ride to build up to an intense and longer-lasting climax.

★ Take note of how long it takes for you to bring your girl to digital climax and how long it takes to bring her to orgasm using a pocket rocket. Notice the moves that bring her over the top. Experiment with the vibrator going in circles, back and forth, and up and down. Digital play is a great technique to master so you can find opportunities to turn any date into a sexy party.

THE LEAD-IN

Tell her the weather report and ski conditions that morning and make a promise to keep her warm. Follow it up with a wink of an eye and a pat on the butt.

THE FOREPLAY

① Set her barometer for hot before you hit the slopes. Begin by kissing her neck, breasts, and waist all the way down to her vulva. When you get there, let out a warm breath.

② Feather your tongue over her clit so she knows she can feel something, but make it so soft that it is almost ticklish.

③ Apply some warming lube on and around her clit with your finger. This will increase sensitivity and give her a nice start to her day. Better than an energy drink.

④ When you get into the gondola ride, open the hand warmer and ask your snow bunny to sit in your lap, warm her hands, and enjoy the view with you.

⑤ Kiss and blow a warm breath on her neck. Go for some outercourse. Grab her hips and thrust your penis against her butt, sparking a fire from all the friction. Mmmmm.

★ The Main Act

1. Add the warming lube to your fingers, unbutton and unzip her pants, reach your hand in, move her panties aside, and apply.

2. If you are right-handed, position her on your right knee for increased dexterity. This will also give you the option to pull out your penis for easy stroking with your left hand or hers.

3. Start with a gentle touch that caresses the inner walls of each of her labia.

4. Move up to the commissure, then rub it with slightly more pressure than you would the clitoris.

5. Speaking of clitoral delights, move down to the clitoris. You are going to give indirect clitoral stimulation.

6. Cover the clitoris with the labia and apply indirect rubs, using her outer lips to stimulate the clit. Next, take the same concept up a notch and place your middle finger against one outer labia and the pointer finger on the other outer labia, gently squeeze your fingers, and move them in opposing directions. This feels incredible and you will look like a pro.

7. Alternate the labia-stroking technique with some gentle direct strokes to the clit. If it is a tight fit in her pants your hand may be pushed on the clitoris, creating too much direct stimulation. Instead, push her pants out with the knuckles of your fist, so your finger can move freely and *gently* over her clitoris. This is very important to the move. Too much pressure on the clit when she is not yet aroused enough can be painful.

8. Pay attention to what she is doing, too. Is she moaning with pleasure, scooting away in pain, or rolling around in your lap in ecstasy?

9. On the last run of the day, pull out the pocket rocket and do the sequence you know works best. To avoid overstimulation, start with different kinds of light stimulation and leave the vibrator for the end.

10. When you find her sweet spot, stick with it. Ask her to tell you when she is coming. When you hear those sweet words, pause and cease sensation, reapply the vibe for a surge of vibrator stimulation, and watch her reawaken with one of the most electrifying and longest orgasms she's ever had.

11. Pull out the warming gel whenever she needs a reminder that you know how to keep things hot in below-freezing temperatures.

RELATED MOVES

★ Sit beside her and lay down a jacket. From this position, you can reach for her hand and put it in your pants for a nice warm-up hand job or mutual hand job.

♀ WHY IT WORKS FOR HER

★ Small amounts of clitoral stimulation over a long period of time help build the tension—and result in an intense, long-lasting orgasm.

★ If the cool mountain air and snowy scenery don't make her feel fresh and alive, the vibrating jolt will!

♂ WHY IT WORKS FOR HIM

★ Dry humping brings back memories of the early days when that was as far as you got. Wasn't it exciting? Now see what it does for your downhill skiing.

|||||||||||||||||||||||||||||||||||||||||||||||||||||||||||||||||||||||||||||||||||||||||||||||||||||||||||||||||||||

THE SEXPERT SAYS

Generally speaking, one of the major differences between how men and women approach sex is that men tend to be more orgasm focused. This can cause performance anxiety and possibly an inability to orgasm for women. Remember, this is for her. Learn to savor the touch that doesn't lead to immediate orgasm, be in the moment, and enjoy each of the phases of the sexual response cycle for what it is.

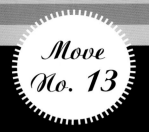

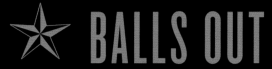 BALLS OUT

Exercise balls are so fun and ultra hot. Have your girl lie on the ball so it rests between her lower and upper back, as if she were going to do sit ups. You rest on your knees with her feet resting on your thighs. You hold on to her breasts and pull her in and out, all the while twisting her nipples.

The Move: Balls Out

THE PREPARATIONS

★ Fill the ball with air.

★ Unless you have used the exercise ball for sex before, you will want to practice going through these steps while maintaining good balance.

THE LEAD-IN

The next time your girl says, "I really need to work out," grab the ball, and tape a large note on it that reads, "Your personal trainer will be here in five minutes. Get naked." Roll the ball out to her. It's okay if she sees you bowling the ball to her in the buck.

THE FOREPLAY

① As her fitness instructor, it is very important that you tell her to stretch. We don't want any accidents.

② Have her lean back on the ball, extending her arms over her head and to the floor into a back bend. This position gives her a stretch and increases blood flow. It also opens her up and makes her ultra vulnerable and accessible. Caress her entire body with your hands.

③ Now it's your turn to stretch. Kneel in front of her vulva. Stretch out your tongue and lap it lustfully over her vulva.

④ And, would you look at that, she is in the perfect position to fellate you, her instructor. That is very naughty. Even better, her head is positioned at the perfect tilt for deep throating you.

THE SEXPERT SAYS

We would probably be very well served if we looked silly in front of our partners within the first few minutes of meeting. Now that that's over, we can all relax, have fun, and be ourselves. This is one silly move that will help you get over those initial jitters.

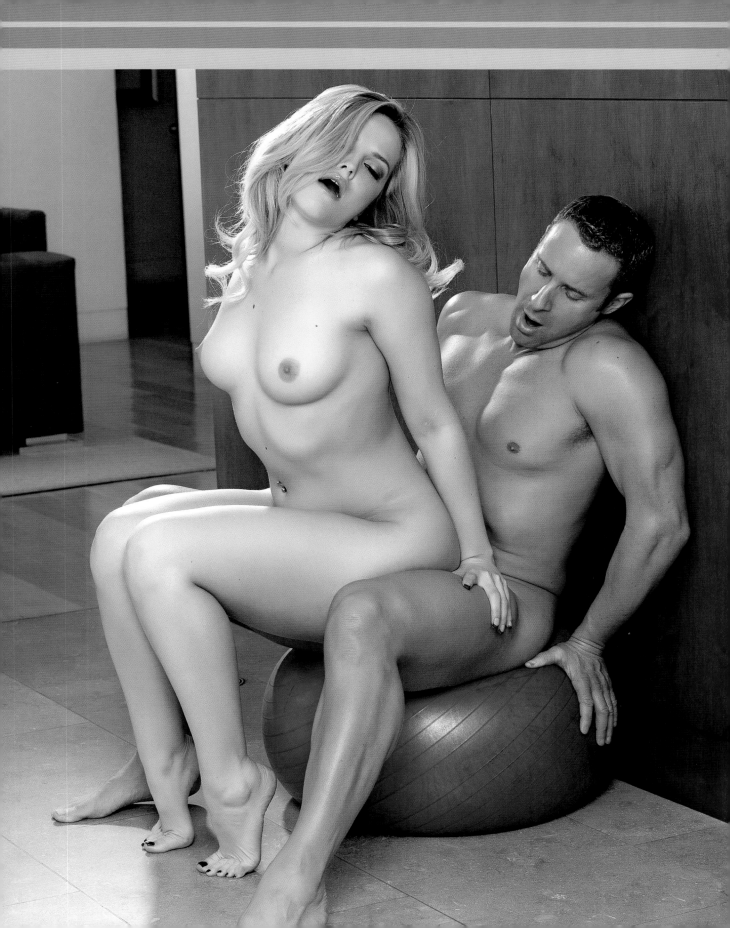

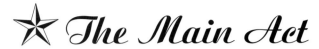 The Main Act

1 Have her scoot forward so her feet are flat on the floor; the ball should slide closer to her upper back and support her head.

2 Kneel in front of her and insert your penis into her vagina so her feet are resting on your thighs. Hold on to her breasts and pull her in and out as you twist her nipples.

3 Thrust slowly and steadily and be sure not to pump too hard or too fast. She can also control the depth of penetration by offering resistance and pressing her heels to the ground.

4 Have her turn over onto her belly where you can now penetrate her from behind. Hold on to the sides of the ball and pull it into you for depth and control. (See above right.)

5 Now it's your turn for a seat. This position requires more communication and a bit more balance from both of you, which is great for building muscle. Push the ball up against the wall and sit down so the wall is like the back of the chair. Press your feet back to offer resistance and invite her to sit on your lap and hold on to your shoulders while you support her back and pull her in close to lick her neck and nipples. With her feet touching the ground, she can now initiate a slow bounce, riding your cock like one of those masturbation balls with a dildo attached to one end. That's you, her human sex toy bouncing to the beat and to orgasm.

RELATED MOVES

★ Have her sit on your lap with her back facing you. (See below right.) You can feel a little freer in this position because she can offer more resistance and control by pushing off her feet; there's also less risk of her falling backward. Have her lean forward, stretched out on her stomach. You can reach around and digitally manipulate her clitoris and bury your face in her rear for a little butt kissing.

♀ WHY IT WORKS FOR HER

★ This position tilts her pelvis up, allowing for a lot of clitoral stimulation.

★ She will enjoy watching you work extra hard to balance her on the ball and slip your penis in her vagina.

♂ WHY IT WORKS FOR HIM

★ Once you are able to work the balance and manage the movement, you will love the deep penetration it offers and the ability to rub her clit.

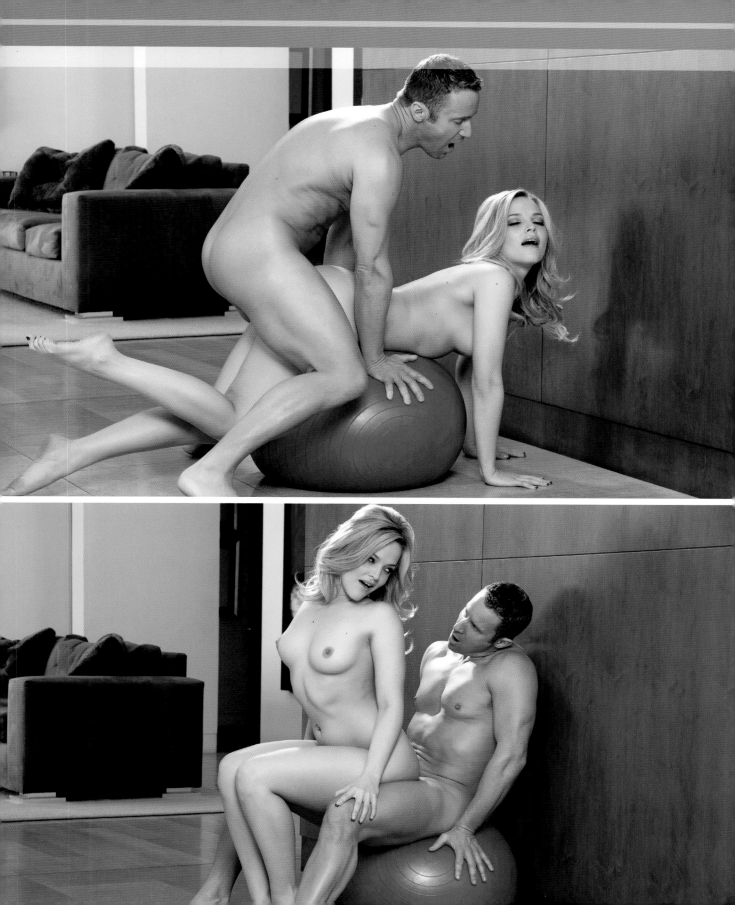

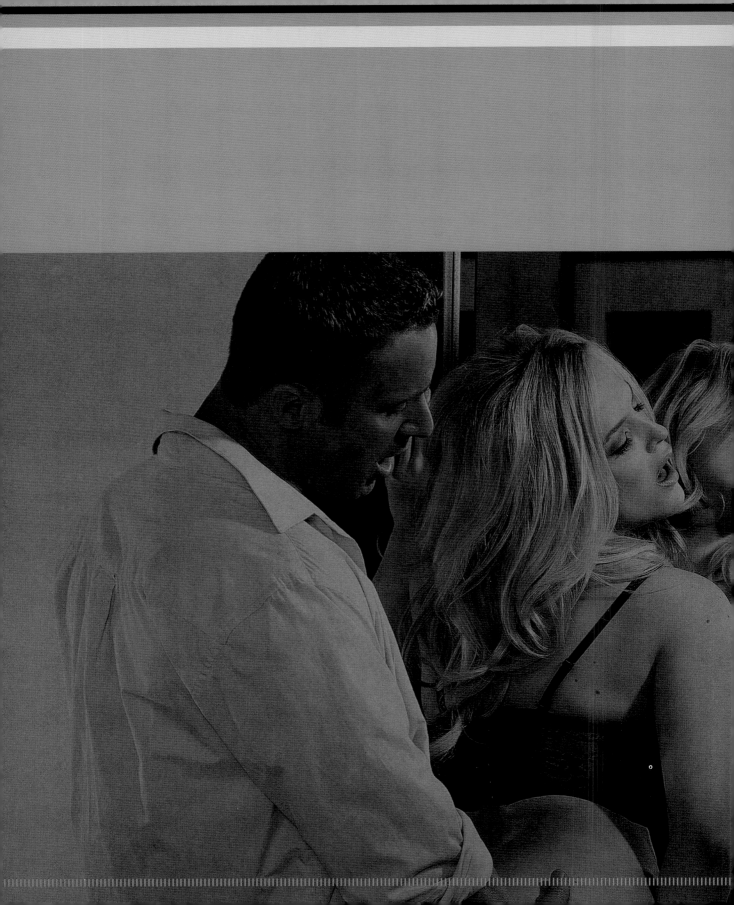

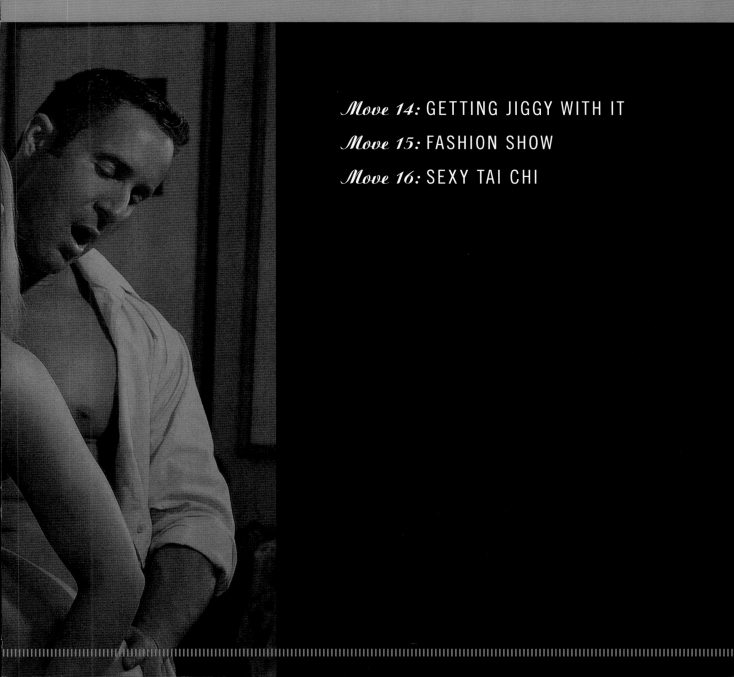

Standing

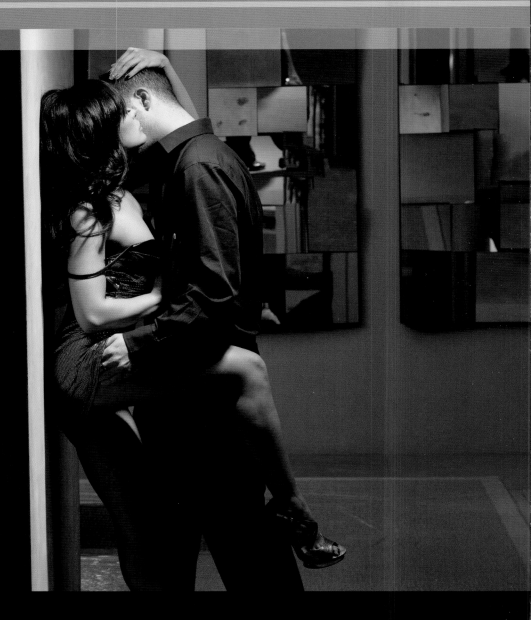

 # GETTING JIGGY <u>WITH</u> IT

Dancing is at the top of almost every woman's fantasy list, while sex is at the top of yours. Bring your list and her list together and get jiggy with it in the corner of a dark dance club or your home disco. You don't have to be Patrick Swayze for this scenario to work, but you will get to try positions that no one saw on the screen!

The Move: Getting Jiggy with It

THE PREPARATIONS

★ Choose some dance music and clothes that make you feel sexy.

★ Scope out dance clubs for dark corners, or turn your place into an instant disco with a black lightbulb.

★ Play some music and practice grinding your hips. Put your hands out in front of you as if you were going to have sex standing up to the music (ultimately you will). Move in circles, to the front, side, and back. Do what moves you. Avoid the desire to be perfect and just have fun. If you are not smiling, you are too caught up in performing.

★ Hold your own eye contact in the mirror as you dance without breaking the glance. It's a game. If you break the eye contact, you lose. You lose the connection and the chance to turn this dance sexy. For red-hot dance communication, hold your eye contact and imagine that you are communicating your sexual desires nonverbally with the music.

THE LEAD-IN

Make her a CD with some of your favorite songs. Write an invitation that says, "I will pick you up at 9 p.m. on Saturday night to go dancing. Wear a long skirt and no panties." Give the CD invitation to her early in the week.

THE FOREPLAY

① Make your entrance into the dance club holding hands. Celebrate her and give her your energy with touch, eye contact, and words. Tell her how stunning she looks throughout the night. She likely spent hours getting dressed up and beautiful for *you*. You can't overdo this.

② If you want an amazingly erotic evening where she feels beautiful, sexy, and free, do *not* indulge yourself by looking at other women when you are with her. Do it behind dark glasses, when you are watching TV at home, or when you are out with your buddies, but not with her. The exception, of course, is if she feels turned on by you looking at other women.

③ Buy her a drink. While at the bar, send her your sexy passion through a smoldering kiss. Kiss her on the lips, neck, shoulders, and chest.

④ Shimmy your way to the dance floor. Spin her. Turn her by her waist.

⑤ Turn up the heat with some nostalgic erotic touch, by putting your hands on her butt and holding her real close like you did with those girls in high school.

⑥ Bump and grind her from behind. Turn her so the front of your body is pressed against her backside. Put your hands on her thighs and thrust your cock against her ass.

7. Turn her around and melt her with your eyes. Dip her. While you look her in the eye, make like you are going to give her a passionate kiss and then tease her by changing positions, returning her to standing.

8. Now bring her real close so she can feel your breath and your sweat. Do the front grind and let your hard cock rub up against her leg, pubic bone, and clitoris, dancing around her pussy.

★ The Main Act

1. Take her to a dark corner of the club and position her with her back to the wall. You are standing face to face with your bodies touching. Wrap your arms around her as if giving her a hug. This will provide support and a tight embrace so no one can see.

2. Lift up her skirt to cover your pants and pull out your cock from the zipper opening. Spread your legs and bend your knees so the head of your cock is below her vulva.

3. Extend your legs slowly to a stand-up position, keeping her close, licking her breasts and neck as you come up.

4. When your cock gets to her vulva, put your hands on her butt and pull her onto your cock, penetrating her.

5. Bump and grind at half the speed. Slower is sexier.

6. Kiss and bite her neck as you bump and grind. Stroke her hair and describe how good it feels to be inside of her.

7. Lift one of her legs, put your hands on her ass, and do more bumping and grinding. This will give even deeper penetration.

8. Contract your PC muscle and see if she can feel you dancing inside her. Find a rhythm and position that she likes and keep that going until orgasm.

||||||||||||||||||||||||||||||||||||||||||||||||||||||||||||||||||||||||||||||||||||||||||||||||||||||||||||||||||||

THE SEXPERT SAYS

Sex is like dancing, flowing with each other in movement. Sex is also like dancing in that if we are focused on the performance, we are not only ineffective, but we are also not having as much fun as we could be.

9. While she is climaxing, hold her close and maintain the speed, rhythm, and pattern as you jiggy through each orgasmic contraction.

10. Continue the embrace, swaying and slow dancing toward resolution.

11. Play the invitation CD every once in a while for a dance, a good laugh, or simply to cheer yourselves up. See whether she has a positive sexual response when she hears the first song.

RELATED MOVES

★ Keep her in high arousal all night and take the last dance to the car. Have her sit spread-eagle in the center of the car, and lace her feet in the seatbelts to do The Slinging Dixie from my book *Spectacular Sex Moves He'll Never Forget*.

♀ WHY IT WORKS FOR HER

★ Dancing and having sex in public is an erotic combo for many people. If she is highly orgasmic and highly aroused, she may have her first climax during the bump and grind with her clothes on.

★ Dancing together increases the heart rate and relaxes the muscles in the pelvis (the erotic center) while thrusting rubs her clitoris.

♂ WHY IT WORKS FOR HIM

★ You'll experience full-on friction to the whole penis and fantastic sensations to the head of your cock when you lift her legs.

★ All your seduction and outercourse may bring on nostalgia for your high school prom days.

||||||||||||||||||||||||||||||||||||||||||||||||||||||||||||||||||||||||||||||||||||||||||||||||||||||||||||||

SEX FACT

The Sydney Morning Herald reported a study that found that men with the best dance moves have the most sex appeal.

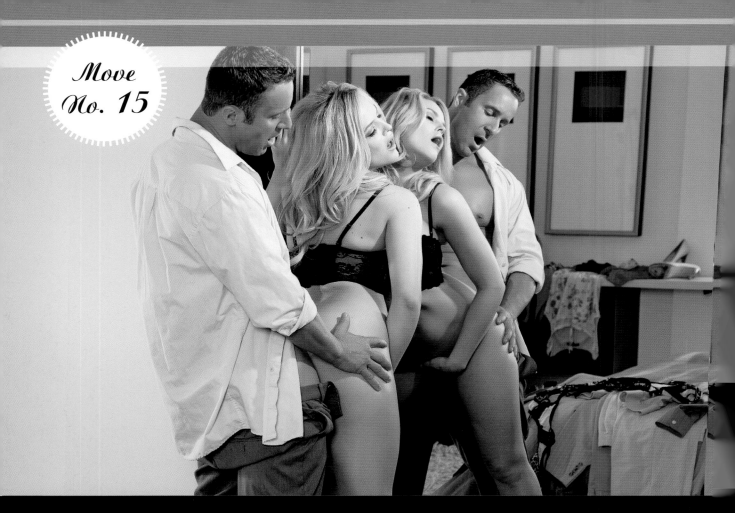

 # FASHION SHOW

Sorry, but it is true: shopping is highly arousing for some women. This scenario is a fashionable way to present your lovely lady with gifts for a special occasion. Or have her model what she's bought while you drive her crazy with your sex moves, one article of clothing at a time.

Women love to hear what you are thinking and how you feel about them, particularly after sex. Sometimes they will ask/demand that you tell them. This is usually a sure sign that you are not expressing enough. Tell her *before* she has to ask. In this move, you will learn to address the "Does my butt look big in these jeans?" question and get to share in the joy of adorning her as you truthfully express what you appreciate about her. Don't miss this

The Move: Fashion Show

THE PREPARATIONS

★ The next time you see a piece of her clothing or shoes, notice the size and the brand. This simple observation of what she likes will help you make decisions and demonstrate your thoughtfulness. Thoughtfulness is romance and what fuels her fire.

★ If you can afford it, buy her an entire sexy outfit, including jewelry, dress, and shoes. If not, hop on the opportunity when she brings home that big bag of clothes.

★ Locate a full-length mirror, and clear out a space in front of it so she has enough room to strut her stuff.

THE LEAD-IN

Sit down, turn on some music, get comfortable, and ask her to model her new outfit. When she says, "What are you talking about?" hand her the package with the jewelry. Watch her open it and tell her what made you think of her when you got the present. Ask her to go try it on.

THE FOREPLAY

① When she comes out, encourage her with your smile. Stand up, grab her hand, and take her to the mirror. Have her look in the mirror as you tell her something truthful and positive about the anatomy you adore as you nuzzle her neck and nibble on that sparkly jewelry. Tell her what made you think of her when you bought the gift. Remember, it's about the thought, so what were you thinking?

② Hand her the box with the dress and say, "You need something to wear that with." Send her off to try it on.

③ The moment she walks out she is going to be reading your face to see whether you really like it. Give her a smile, walk her to the mirror, and tell her what you like about how it adorns her already beautiful body; she can watch as you massage her breasts and gently tweak her nipples between your thumb and forefinger. Rub your cock against her backside and let her feel your hardness.

④ Scratch your head and explain that something is missing. Hand her the shoebox.

⑤ She is getting the hang of this now. When she comes out and turns around, giving you the 360 in her shoes, stand up and give her a passionate kiss.

⑥ Take her to the mirror, get down on your knees, touch her calf, and say, "Those shoes really accent the muscles in your legs. Let's see them without any clothes on . . ."

||||||||||||||||||||||||||||||||||||||||||||||||||||||||||||||||||||||||||||||||||||||||||||||||||||||||||||

SEX FACT

According to Askmen.com, 24.2 percent of women would prefer the gift of designer high heels to oral sex. (How about oral sex in high heels?)

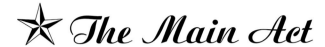

The Main Act

1 Run your hand up her thigh, feeling the heat from her vulva. Have her watch as you remove her dress and bra, saving the panties for last.

2 There's no rush on removing the panties. Nuzzle your face in her crotch, then pull them aside and run your tongue lightly over her pussy; there's something undeniably hot and naughty about teasing and working around clothing. When you're ready, pull, tug, and slide them off with your teeth, removing everything but her jewelry and shoes. A girl needs a little sparkle.

3 You planned this for her without the expectation of reciprocation, but don't be surprised when she wants to suck your cock in gratitude. When she does, have her back facing the mirror. You may never forget the vision of her bending over in heels, her soft rounded breasts rubbing up against you, and her flowering vulva wet and glistening in the reflected light.

4 Stand her up facing the mirror and go down on your knees so she can see you giving her oral sex. Spread her legs and put your finger inside of her and taste her by licking your finger. Tease her with your tongue, feathering her clit to and fro, circling and sucking and giving her oral sex while she stands there in high heels.

5 Stand up and position her so she is leaning against the wall with a hand on each side of the mirror. She is vulnerable with her legs spread, standing and ready to come.

6 Place your hand on her shoulders, lean over, and put your cock inside her with a slow, deep, and hard insertion. Yes!

7 Put one light finger on her clit as you rhythmically pound and stroke her to orgasm in fashion.

8 For a smile, save one of the ribbons and wrap it around your penis the next morning. Recycle the ribbon and make it the gift that keeps on giving.

‖‖‖

SEX FACT

According to a survey by MSNBC/*Elle* magazine, women's top reasons for straying: 44 percent said they were attracted to someone else, and 32 percent said they wanted reassurance of their desirability. (This move gives plenty of reassurance.)

RELATED MOVES

★ Think of this scenario as a great way to give her a gift for her birthday, your anniversary, a holiday, Mother's Day, or just because you want to celebrate her. You can also give her a gift card for her favorite store and ask her to give you a fashion show when she gets home. Or, you can celebrate her without spending the cash. The next time she comes home with some new clothes, have her model each item with something she already has in her closet.

♀ WHY IT WORKS FOR HER

★ Women love words and they love hearing how you feel about them, how you arouse them, and what's on your mind. She probably already knows it, but she wants to hear it and she wants to hear it often. This scenario gives you lots of opportunity for that.

♂ WHY IT WORKS FOR HIM

★ You are going to feel gifted with the vision of her bending over with her long legs in high heels and the reflection of her rear in the mirror.

SEX FACT

According to a survey by MSNBC/*Elle* magazine, 23 percent of women report that feelings about their body make them less interested in having sex.

THE SEXPERT SAYS

Not only does body image keep women from being sexual, but body image issues are also the number one reason a woman cannot climax. Although it's not your responsibility to heal her body image, just like it is not your responsibility to give her an orgasm, a lover who accepts—and appreciates—all of her can really encourage growth and healing in a positive direction.

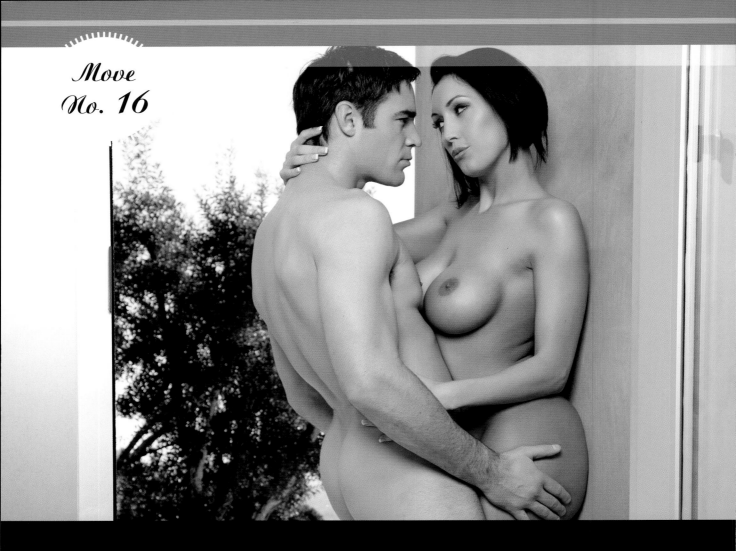

SEXY TAI CHI

A modified version of this exercise is commonly used in martial arts to help train participants to feel their opponent's energy and be in the moment. Movement, energy work, dual meditation, and sex all at the same time make Sexy Tai Chi the perfect position for any occasion.

This is also a great scenario for initiating the arousal phase of the sexual response cycle. The arousal phase is often referred to as the foreplay phase, but all too often it is overlooked. Setting the stage with stimulating scenarios such as this one is perfect for initiating this phase and building up to an intense orgasm for her.

The Move: Sexy Tai Chi

THE PREPARATIONS

★ To learn about energy, get in touch with your own. Close your eyes if you need to and put your arms out in front of you, shoulder-width apart. Slowly move your hands together in front of you. Do you feel the energy? What is it like?

★ Now take a look at her energy. Think of it like a perfume; what is her brand of energy? You may want to ask these questions out loud: Is there a color? Is there a feeling? A taste? A smell? Do you hear something? Wait for an answer. Once you get the information, such as a color, ask what it means. Don't judge it or doubt yourself; simply observe.

★ If you are having trouble identifying her energy, try following each other's energy in a dark room (push the furniture aside) and ask the same questions as above.

★ Text her and let her know you have a surprise for her tonight. Tell her to wear comfortable clothes that make her feel sexy and beautiful.

★ Look around the room. You will want to position her so her back is facing a wall, but standing about 2 feet (61 cm) away so you have that extra space for movement.

THE LEAD-IN

Tonight you are going to be spontaneous. When she walks into the room and sees you doing tai chi to music, take her hands in yours, look into her eyes, and move your hands to the music.

THE FOREPLAY

① Begin the eye gaze by looking at her nondominant eye (usually the left). The left eye is known to be more receptive, more accepting, and less critical. It's also easier to focus on one eye and you won't feel like you are doing an awkward stare down.

② Once you have established eye contact, incorporate conscious breathing. Listen for her breath and notice as her chest rises and falls. Once you find her breath, synchronize your breath with hers. Do this for a few moments and then deepen your own breathing, allowing her to follow you. Subconsciously, this registers for her as trust, connection, and being safely led, or taken.

③ Kiss her neck and slowly remove her clothes while maintaining awareness, being present, and celebrating her beauty with whispers in her ear.

④ Put her hands on your cock and ask her to remove your clothes.

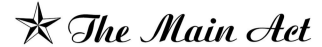

★ The Main Act

1. Maintain the synchronized breathing and eye contact.

2. Standing face to face, reach for her hands and raise them to your chest, with both of your palms touching hers.

3. Move your hands slowly, feeling her energy and allowing her to follow without pattern or expectation. Push your hands backward, then forward, and move them in large circles, small circles, and different directions.

4. Know that you are connected through the hands, but listen to the whole body, the movement, and the breath.

5. Try closing your eyes and take notice of your energy and then hers. Has it changed? How so? Ask her to do the same.

6. Open your eyes. Begin to shift the focus of your movement away from your hands and onto your erotic center. Instead of moving your hands in different circles and directions, move your pelvises. Synch your movements with your breath and flow as one.

7. Adjust your stance by opening your legs wide. Slip your erect cock between her labia and press your pubic bone against her engorged clitoris.

8. Feel her warmth and wetness on the shaft as you move without penetration. Allow yourself to feel her desire for you to enter her.

9. She will be feeling your desire for her, which is extremely hot, *and* she will be feeling her own for you.

10. When both of you are as aroused as possible, guide her so that her back is against the wall. Bend your knees, adjust your stance, look into her eyes, and penetrate.

11. Be one with each other's breath. When you penetrate her, exhale. When she exhales, you inhale, and vice versa.

|||||||||||||||||||||||||||||||||||||||||||||||||||||||||||||||||||||||||||||||||||||||||||||||||||||||||||||||||||||||||||||||

SEX FACT

Music, scents, touches, memories, and behaviors can all serve as positive anchors that can be consciously used to elicit the desired results. One client of mine played the same music each time he had sex (anchor) and now he only needs to hear the first few notes, and boom!—instant erection (desired results).

RELATED MOVES

★ Grab her ass and tilt her pelvis forward. This will give more depth and allow you to grind on her pelvis. Bend and straighten your legs for deeper penetration.

♀ WHY IT WORKS FOR HER

★ She is going to come *fast* because there is a lot of sexual energy exchanged and foreplay makes up about 85 percent of this move. The more time you spend in the arousal phase, the more intense, memorable, and pleasurable the experience will be for her.

♂ WHY IT WORKS FOR HIM

★ You will learn how to create, move, and play with the energy of arousal, in yourself and in her. Most women need and crave a lot of foreplay to climax. Feeling each other's energy is a completely different kind of sex that can lead to more intense, multiple, and longer orgasms.

|||||||||||||||||||||||||||||||||||||||||||||||||||||||||||||||||||||||||||||||||||||||||||||||||||||||||||||||||||||

SEX FACT

Leading with the breath will help establish intimacy and trust and enable you to produce a masculine energy that she can follow.

|||||||||||||||||||||||||||||||||||||||||||||||||||||||||||||||||||||||||||||||||||||||||||||||||||||||||||||||||||||

THE SEXPERT SAYS

You will notice very quickly when you or your partner is "checked out," is in resistance, or is out of the flow. How does going against the flow and offering resistance throw your relationship off balance? Ultimately, with practice, you will both be better at reading and managing the energy and sacred space between you in life and in sex.

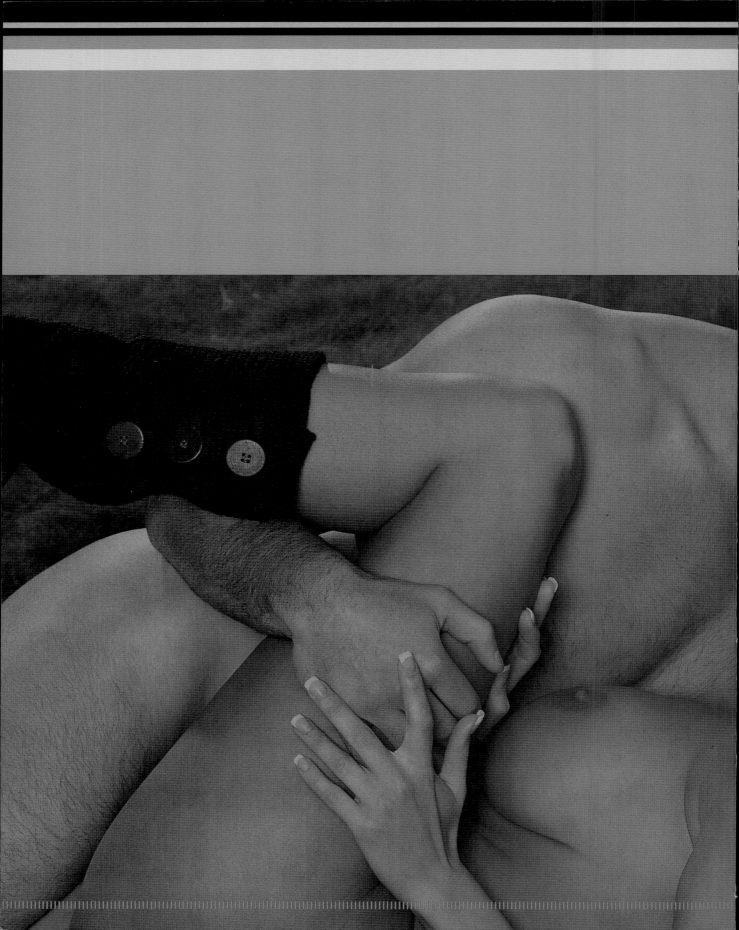

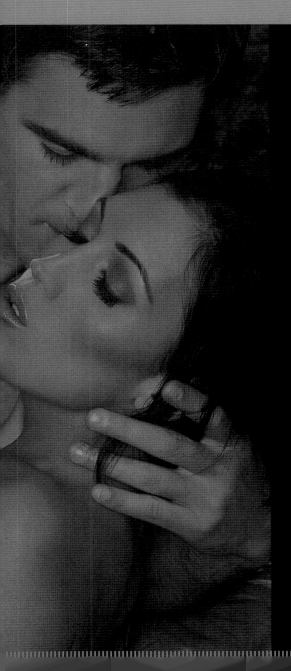

Side by Side

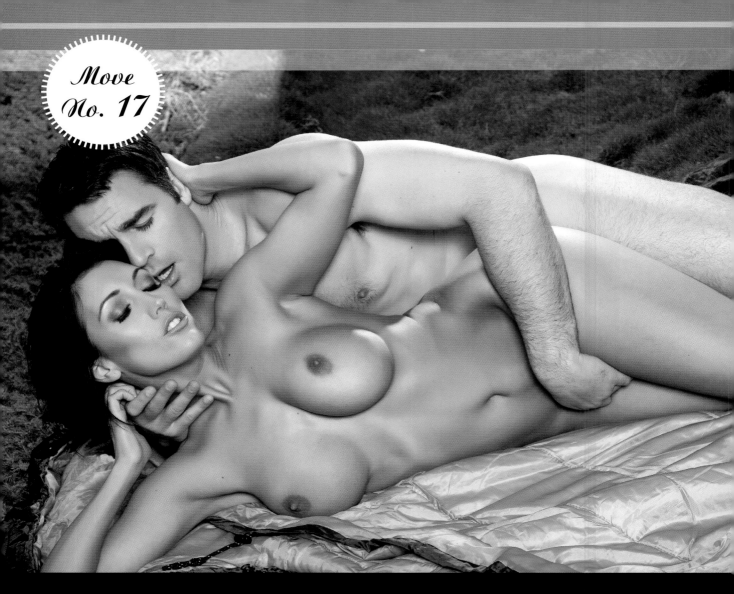

★ REAL CAMPERS <u>DO IT</u> SIDEWAYS

Stars, moonlight, intimacy, and close proximity all wrapped up in one sleeping bag. Use the
constraints of the bag as resistance to move and groove into closer, deeper penetration—all with

The Move: Real Campers Do It Sideways

THE PREPARATIONS

★ A good Boy Scout is always prepared.

★ Pack two sleeping bags for sleeping, but your bag is the one you will invite her into for sex. A mummy bag will not work, although it would be a snug fit for two people and part of the fun.

★ Pack extra towels, baby wipes, and lube for easy gliding.

★ Pack a tarp to lay your bag on for stargazing and sexing. You can carry the bags into the tent later when it is sleeping time. Pack wood, an ax, and a muscle shirt.

★ Surprise her by packing a fun treat, such as s'mores, even if you are not the one planning the food.

★ Don't wait until you are too exhausted to turn in for the night and leave sex for the end. Sex *is* the activity for the night.

★ Let her see you out and about in your muscle shirt, chopping wood and preparing the fire. When you catch her looking, offer a little flex of the muscle. Exaggerate and be playful; this is all in good fun.

★ Start warming her up by kissing her neck and telling her how you can't wait to be with her under the stars.

THE LEAD-IN

While at the fire, make a s'more and feed it to her slowly and sensually. Follow a bite of s'more with a yummy kiss to her sweet lips. Place a little chocolate on your lips or neck and ask her to lick it off.

Invite her into your sleeping bag, where you will be more comfortable.

THE FOREPLAY

① While you are kissing her, pay attention to her nonverbal cues and let her show you her own milky way. If she is exposing her neck or ears, she likely wants you to nibble there; if she brushes her breasts against you, she likely wants you to fondle her breasts; if she is thrusting her pelvis, she likely wants clitoral stimulation; and if she has her hand in your pants, giving your cock long strokes, she probably wants penetration.

② Remove the clothing covering the erogenous zones that are begging to be touched until she is naked.

||||||||||||||||||||||||||||||||||||||||||||||||||||||||||||||||||||||||||||||||||||||||||||||||||||||||||||||||||||||||||||

SEX FACT

ABC News' American Sex Survey reports that 57 percent of Americans have had sex outdoors.

★ The Main Act

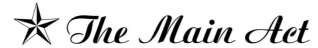

1 Get into the sleeping bag so you are both resting on your elbows in the side-by-side spoon position, your front against her back. Reach the other arm around so you can give long gentle strokes to her breasts. Kiss her neck and shoulders as you slowly penetrate her from behind.

2 Ask her to roll over to her other side so you can face each other. For better clitoral stimulation, continue to rest your weight on your elbows, as you place your arm under her head as a pillow. Lift her top leg to open her up, and place a well-lubed finger on her clitoris. (See near right.)

3 Press your chests and bodies together so you are toe to toe. Lift her top leg again and put it on your waist. Lift and bend your top leg and put it on the inside thigh of her bottom leg. Look into her eyes, pull her close, and slowly insert your cock. (See far right.)

4 She is in the perfect place for some ass play. Massage and knead her butt cheeks, relaxing her. Separate her cheeks and slide your lubed finger over the pucker of her ass. You can use saliva, lube, or vaginal wetness on her ass, but for health reasons, do not go from anus to vagina.

5 Push your feet against the side of the closed sleeping bag for leveraging power and deeper penetration.

6 Tilt your pelvis forward and backward to access all the right spots, finding the spot that feels really good for both of you.

7 Alternatively, have her wrap her leg around your waist (or wrap yours around hers) and offer a directional pull in with the legs and feet.

8 Insert your hand into the perfect amount of space between your bodies for stroking her clitoris. Most women cannot climax without some sort of clitoral stimulation. If she doesn't naturally rub her own clit, do it for her, rubbing all the way to climax.

9 After climax, hold her shoulders and turn on your back so she is on top of you. Marvel at the magic of the universe and count your lucky stars.

RELATED MOVES

★ Unzip the bag all the way open and go down to the opposite end of the bag. Both of you should lie on your sides, intertwined. She rests her head on your foot as you hold her hands and pull her into you. You massage her rear and thighs while she massages your testicles and feet. This is a side-to-side position with a new angle.

SEX FACT

Dasofallation is sexual intercourse in a forest or wooded area.

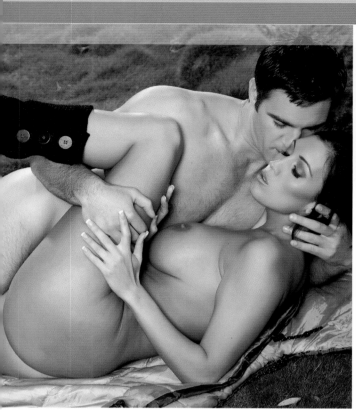
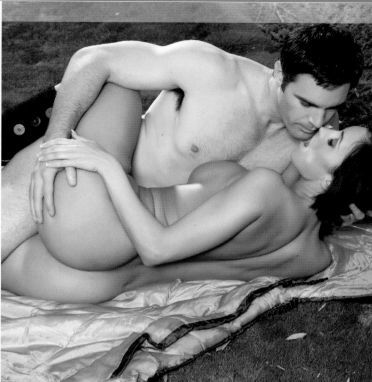

♀ WHY IT WORKS FOR HER

★ It is very, very sexy to see men in their natural element of the great outdoors, chopping wood in a muscle shirt. This position gives that skin-to-skin, muscle-to-clit, and muscle-to-tit contact she has been dreaming about.

♂ WHY IT WORKS FOR HIM

★ Being romantic and being her star has never been easier with this position. You will love the dynamics the sleeping bag offers for leverage, so you have more control to hit all the right spots on your cock.

||||||||||||||||||||||||||||||||||||||||||||||||||||||||||||||||||||||||||||||||||||||||||||||||||||||||||||||||||||||

THE SEXPERT SAYS

Don't mistake a "great lover" with a performer, or someone who has all the moves and techniques but none of the supporting qualities. Being a great performer will only take you so far. A great lover has excellent technique but first and foremost is thoughtful, patient, and observant, and makes a woman feel cared for, adored, and special.

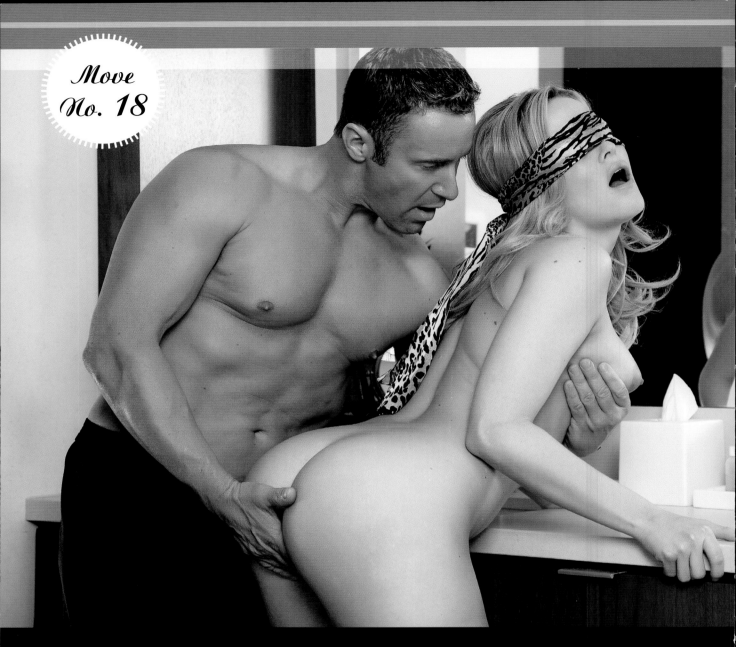

Move
No. 18

PLEASURE PARTY

This may be the closest you get to group sex. She is lying on her side, blindfolded, as you penetrate her with your cock, one hand stimulating her nipples, your mouth kissing her shoulders, and whispering an erotic story in her ear, while a dildo in her ass makes the perfect pleasure party for two!

The Move: Pleasure Party

THE PREPARATIONS

★ Talk about your fantasies ahead of time and keep it close in your mental database.

★ Some women might have a multiple person fantasy. If so, how many? Is hers male, female, both, or an orgy?

★ Sometimes fantasies come at the darnedest times, such as in a meeting or during a drive to work. If you can entertain the fantasy at the time, great! Otherwise, take note of it and revisit it when you get a chance. You can also watch porn to see what arouses you.

★ Position some lube, a blindfold, Nipple Nibblers cream, clamps or clothespins, and her favorite anal dildo or vibrating dildo nearby.

★ If this is your first time doing anal with your partner, make sure you discuss it ahead of time and verify that she's interested. Also, if you are going to use a vaginal toy in the anus, use a separate anal toy. I always suggest using a condom on the dildo because most sex toys are porous and very difficult to clean. Bacteria from the anus can cause nasty infections in the vagina.

THE LEAD-IN

Wrap the blindfold around her eyes as you whisper in her ear and describe the special guests coming over that night. Lead her to the bed and lay her down on her side.

THE FOREPLAY

① Lie down beside her and kiss her shoulders. Approaching from the rear gives a different angle. Stimulate her erotic mind and ask her who she wants to come to the party. Ask her to describe the person: What would he or she look like? How would the person hear about the party? How would the party happen?

② As she describes the fantasy, suckle her nipples. Put a clothespin on them to hold the stimulation while you explore other areas. The pinch will feel good, but also increase nipple sensitivity in general.

③ Gently bite and kiss her neck. Glide your hand up her thighs and slip your finger in between her lips. Feel her wetness and softly rub the clitoral shaft, then move gently over the clitoral glans.

④ Ask her to talk about the fantasy as you go down and give her oral to orgasm. The clitoral orgasm will relax all her muscles, including her sphincter, so she can more comfortably receive anal from the fantasy partner.

SEX FACT

Askmen.com reports that a threesome is in the top ten of female fantasies. According to ABC News' American Sex Survey, 8 percent of women have participated in a threesome. More women have fantasized about a threesome than have actually participated in one.

★ The Main Act

1 Lie down sideways, facing each other. Begin kissing her while she is blindfolded and start narrating the story.

2 Spread her butt cheeks and glide your finger over the sphincter. Using a well-lubed finger, gently press down on the pucker of the anus; if she is relaxed enough, your finger should easily glide in. Replace your finger with a dildo.

3 Start off by slowly pressing the dildo, slowly twirling it, and slowly pushing it in and out, paying close attention to what she likes. (See above right.) While holding one hand on the dildo, suckle and blow cool air on her clothespin-pinched nipples.

4 Ask her which one of her characters is going to fuck her pussy? As she talks, insert your cock deep inside of her. Gently grab her ass and bring her close, giving her slow, deep thrusts with your cock and slow rhythmic penetrations from the dildo so she is receiving from both ends. (See below right.)

5 Orchestrate the fucking, sucking, and dildo-bucking pleasure party.

RELATED MOVES

★ Use your own tools to penetrate her in multiple places. Have her lean over a table and rest on her hands so she is arm's distance away from the table. Get on your knees and lick her vulva; one hand can reach for her breast and twist her nipples. With the other hand, put your thumb on her G-spot and your middle finger up her ass. Now that's a party!

♀ WHY IT WORKS FOR HER

★ The side-by-side position (and blindfold) allows her mind to run free with the fantasy. The foreplay orgasm will help relax her sphincter muscles, making penetration easier.

★ The vaginal and anal penetration combination adds to the pressure and feelings of fullness that women crave. Also, stimulating the nipples while penetrating her can amp up the sensation and oftentimes bring her over the top.

♂ WHY IT WORKS FOR HIM

★ There is a great deal of variety to play with in this position. Also, inserting a dildo into the anus narrows the vaginal canal, allowing for a tighter grip on the penis.

|||||||||||||||||||||||||||||||||||||||||||||||||||||||||||||||||||||||||||||||||||||||||||||||||||||||||||||||||

THE SEXPERT SAYS

Fantasies and daydreaming can bring us a lot of safe pleasure. Just because we have fantasies doesn't mean that we necessarily want to act them out. Some people simply like the idea more than the act.

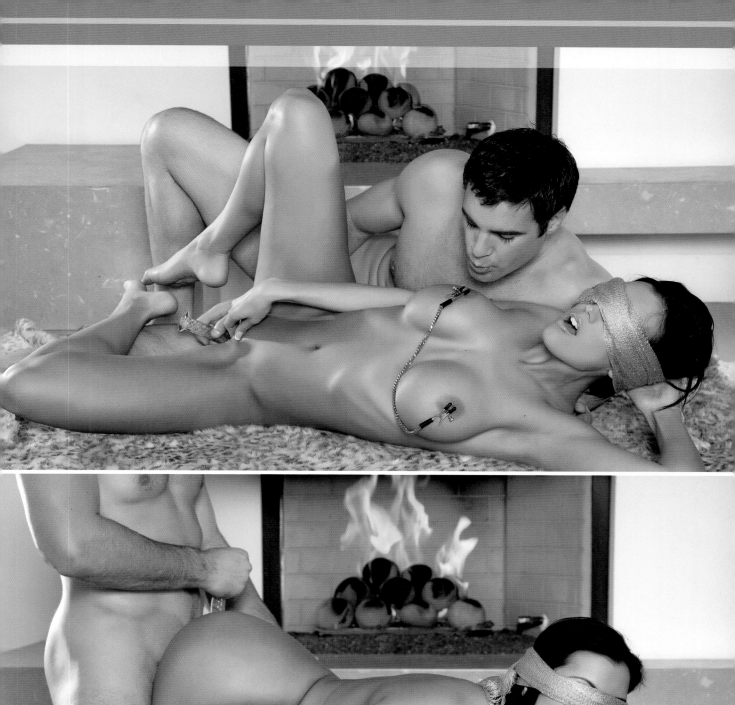
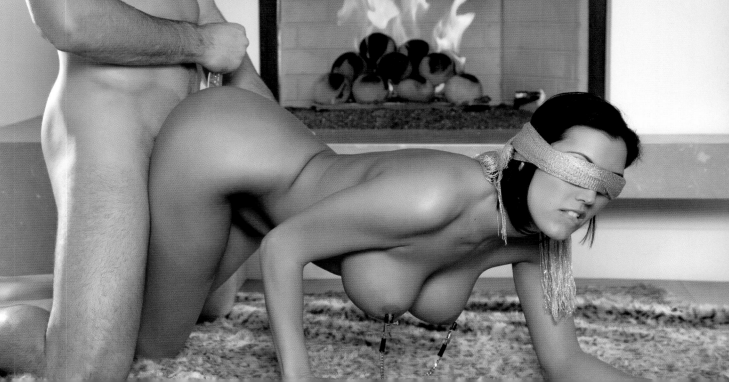

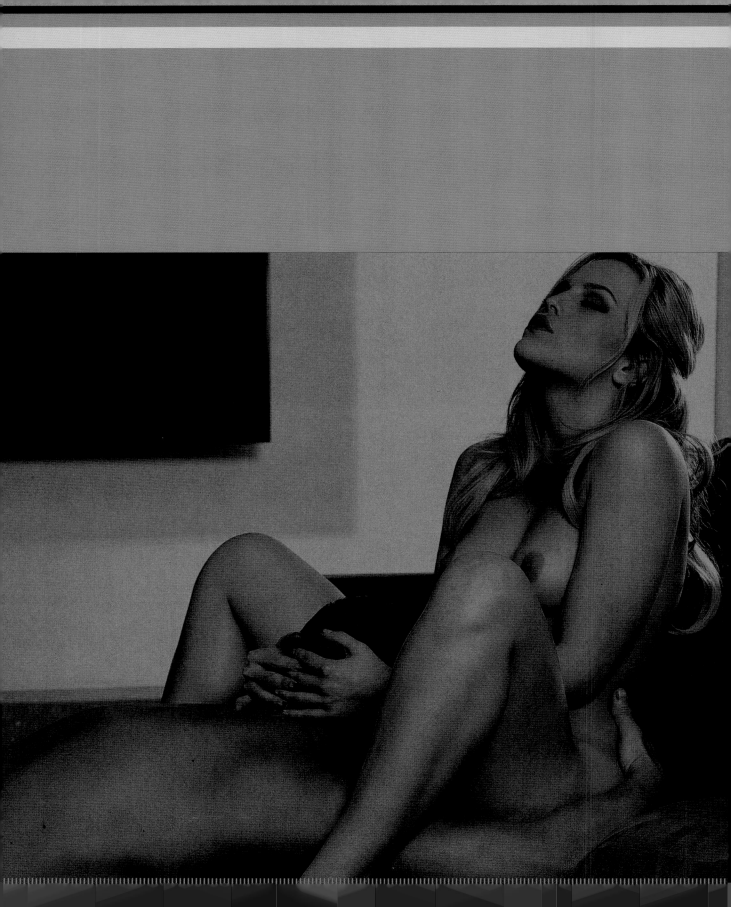

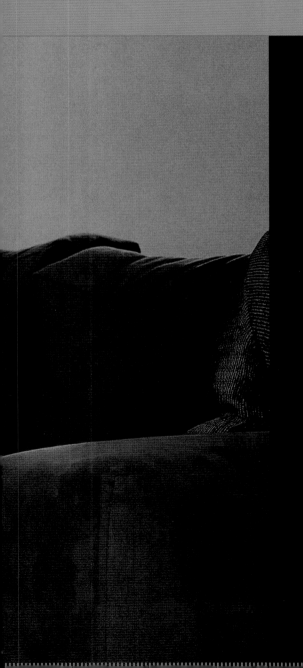

Oral Sex

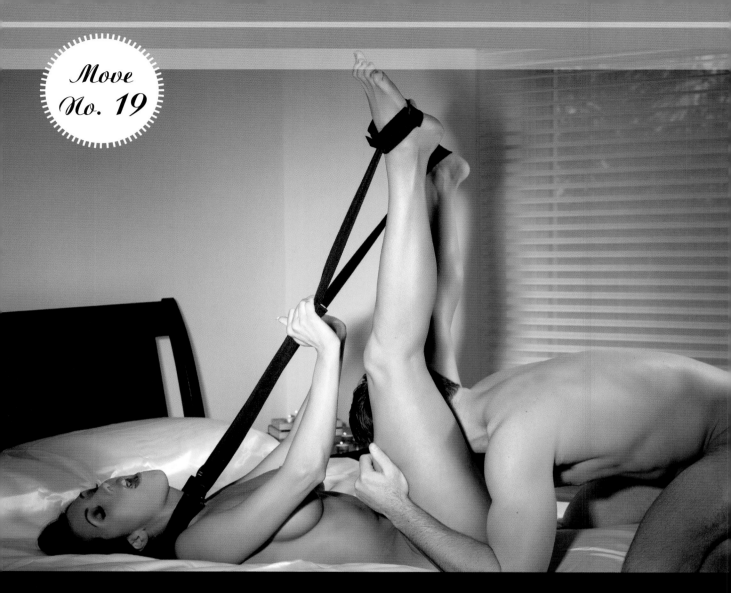

 # SHAGALICIOUS

Satin sheets, candles, rose petals, and her legs spread open in an oral sex sling means all she has to do is enjoy as you give her U-spot stimulation and the most luscious orgasm she has ever had. This is unconditional giving at its best and it's better than any spa or prescription; it's what a woman secretly wants from a massage—one with a release.

You probably already know this by now, but when it comes to romance, it really is the thought that counts and it counts *big*, whether you have cash or not.

The Move: Shagalicious

THE PREPARATIONS

★ Make the bed shag ready with satiny sheets, candles, rose petals, feathers, body oil, and chocolate.

★ Make an ankle sex sling: tie three or four neckties together. They will ultimately be tied around both of her ankles and slung over your back so she doesn't exert any effort to even hold her legs up.

★ Clean the tub and run a bubble bath, playing soft music.

★ Meditate on her beauty and your gratitude for her. Intention always shows up, whether it's in your face, gestures, or touch.

THE LEAD-IN

Flowers are in order. Send her flowers or leave a message for her that says, "Hello, beautiful. I have a sexy spa day waiting for you when you get home. Everything is ready. Come as you are."

When she gets home, take her to the bubble bath and tell her to come out when she is ready.

THE FOREPLAY

① Lay her belly down on the satiny sheets. Delight her with light, gentle strokes to her back and whole body with the feather, then your hands. Do this without oil and be sure to include the ears, scalp, and feet.

② Set the intention for loving/caring. Feel your fingertips against her skin; feel the softness and firmness in her body. Make love with your hands and feel her whole being, letting it inspire and arouse you. If in doubt, go lighter.

③ Turn her over, offer her some chocolate, and give the same long, slow strokes to her front side with the feather, then with the oil.

④ Start from the feet and work your way up, sensually separating her thighs. Glide your fingers over her mons and through her pubic hair. Slide each of her labia between well-lubed fingers as if gently pinching, and move your way up, giving each your undivided attention.

THE SEXPERT SAYS

Touch is a very important part of communication. Women sometimes comment that their partner only touches them when they want to be sexual. Make sure that a large portion of your touch is nonsexual. Set your intention through your touch and let her find her arousal through the process. Examples of nonsexual touch include massage, hand holding, love pats, kisses, and general nurturing.

(5)   Separate the labia, using your pointer finger and thumb, then massage up and down along the sides of the clitoral shaft. Do the same with the top of the clitoral shaft, leaving out the clitoral glans.

(6)   Use your pointer and middle fingers to move in a figure eight, starting at the commissure, down and across the urethra, or U-spot, and then down and around the base of the vaginal opening. Do this a few times and then change directions, keeping the same pattern.

(7)   Insert your pointer and middle fingers into her vagina and press up toward her navel, pressing on the G-spot while you gently rub your thumb over the clitoris.

(8)   Incorporate the genital massage with the whole body by moving your free hand over the abdomen, then breasts, then shoulders.

★ The Main Act

1   Lay her on her back and wrap the sling around each ankle. An ankle sling is shagalicious because she doesn't even have to put out effort to hold her legs up. Once you have her in the sling, you can rest it on your shoulders or other parts of your body and have your hands free.

2   Push the sling back, raising and exposing her entire rear end. Lick all of her with a sloppy, wet, flat tongue, and cover the entire surface area.

3   Gently suck on the clitoris and repeat the same pattern that you did with your fingers, but with your pointed tongue: move in a figure eight, starting at the commissure, down and across the urethra, or U-spot, and then down and around the base of the vaginal opening. Do this a few times and then change directions, keeping the same pattern.

4   Listen for her breath. When she inhales and exhales deeply, she is relaxed.

5   Insert your pointer and index fingers into her vagina and press up toward her navel, pressing on the G-spot. When you're ready for her to climax, continue to stimulate her G-spot as you press your gums on her commissure, then place your puckered lips over her clitoris as you suckle and twirl your tongue to a very happy ending.

6   Continue to stroke her throughout resolution, with long, soft strokes of your hand and the feather while you feed her chocolate.

SEX FACT

When asked about his favorite part of the vulva, Ian Kerner, author of *She Comes First*, answered: "They're all wonderful in their own unique way. . . . But . . . if I had to pick one, I'd say the front commissure."

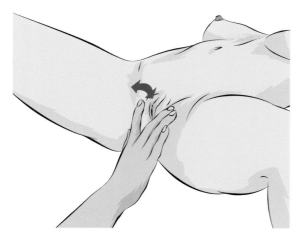

Separate the labia and massage up and down along the sides of the clitorial shaft.

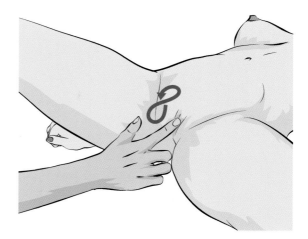

Move your finger in a figure eight starting at the commissure, down and across the urethia, and then down around the base of the vaginal opening.

RELATED MOVES

★ Remove one of her ankles from the sling, so only one is tied. Maneuver her tied ankle with the length of the sling, or give it to her to manage as she wishes. This will make for a completely different feeling in the position.

★ The ankle sling can also be adjusted and used as handcuffs or a light bondage device for positions of surrender.

♀ WHY IT WORKS FOR HER

★ Passively receiving in total relaxation makes this position a true gift, and when woman are relaxed, they are more orgasmic.

★ This combination of genital massage and oral stimulation with many of the hot spots (G-spot, U-spot, and pressure on the commissure) is off the charts.

♂ WHY IT WORKS FOR HIM

★ You will appreciate how easy it is to maneuver her into position and tap into the spots that are good for you and her, while having your hands free to touch her or yourself. Ultra hot.

★ The genital massage gives you lots of practice stimulating many of her hot spots, first with your hands and then later with your mouth.

SEX FACT

Men are more likely to consider the onset of sex to be the moment of penetration, but women see the tease, kissing, and foreplay as part of the overall sexual experience.

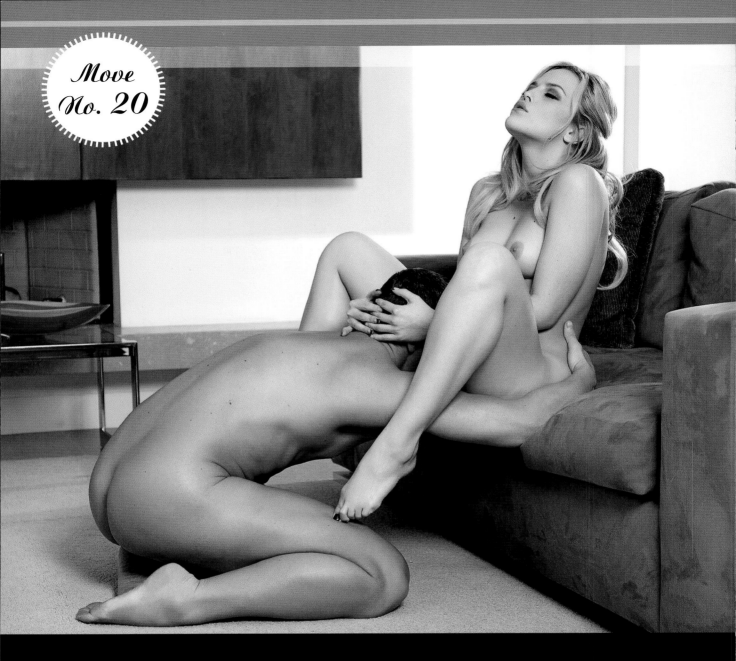

THE KISS OF DATE

Take her on a lusty, adventurous kissing date where passionate kisses abound and she can't wait for you to bring that kiss farther, farther, and farther down south until you taste her sexiness.

The Move: The Kiss of Date

THE PREPARATIONS

★ The secret to sensuality with a woman is in the kiss. In preparation for your kiss of date, imagine that the only way you can communicate to her is through your kiss. If your kiss were to communicate for you without words, what would you say?

★ Shave your face free of stubbles and cut your nails. Nothing ruins an oral sex moment like whiskers and hangnails. Have water and breath mints handy for you and her. Get moist with some lip balm.

★ Pay attention to your kissing. How do you kiss? Practice your kisses in your mind and or on your hand. Consider these elements when kissing: Where are you kissing her? Do you use an open mouth or a closed mouth? Do you do nibbles or pecks? Do your kisses involve a licking trailer? Are they wet or dry? Do you use tongue and if so, how?

★ How is your body positioned when you kiss her? Do you use flavored lip balm? Do you have fresh breath? Is it a surprise kiss? Are your eyes open or closed? Do you add a little suction?

THE LEAD-IN

Send her a fun card for no reason except to tell her that you think she is amazing and to announce your date for the weekend: "I will pick you up at 7 p.m. on Saturday for our date. I can't wait to kiss your sweet lips." If you know she likes Brazilian waxes, get a gift certificate from her favorite salon and put it in the envelope.

THE FOREPLAY

① As soon as she answers the door, kiss her passionately as if you have been waiting your whole life to kiss her. Close your eyes and kiss her as if she is the only thing in your mind and heart at that given moment.

② Open your mouth and kiss her with puckered, moist lips, and a soothing tongue that traces hers. Breathe in and out through your nose, smelling her smell and letting her smell your fresh breath.

③ On the release, slowly break away only to come back for more. Switch the position of your head for comfort, yours and hers. Hold her gaze as you rub noses and brush lips.

④ Kiss her in a series of quick pecks with relaxed lips as you move toward the car. Hold some of that yummy energy in your eyes as you look at her and walk to the car to open her door.

SEX FACT

Taoists believe that the lips, tongue, fingers, and genitals are a few of the main channels for exchanging energy.

(5) Before you let her go, take her hand, look into her eyes, and give kisses all the way up her arm, to her neck and ears. Close your eyes and feel her softness against your lips. Let her hear you moan with the pleasure of kissing her.

(6) While at a red light or stop sign, lean over and kiss her neck, her ears, and her cheek. Drive to your favorite romantic restaurant. When you open her car door, reach for her hand and bring her close as if you were going to dance, and then dip her. Kiss her mid-dip with her leg in the air.

(7) Try kissing her with ice cubes between your lips. Offer her a small bite of your food and follow it with a kiss.

(8) All this restaurant entertainment might mean your check will be a long time coming. While you are waiting, kiss with a mint, switching it back and forth in a playful way.

(9) Put your hand in her lap, run your hand up her inner thigh, hold your hand over her vulva, and whisper in her ear, "For dessert."

★ The Main Act

1 Open the car door for her, and offer your hand. As she gets in, look into her eyes as if you were going in for a kiss on the lips, but instead hold the gaze and close the car door. (Gotta have a little anticipation.)

2 Take her inside and slowly undress her. Give her the Kiss of Date undress, where your lips follow your hands, kissing the newly exposed and unclothed flesh.

3 Position her on your bed or a nest of soft blankets on the floor. Starting with her feet, kiss, lick, and suck her toes. Trail up between her thighs, around her waist, on the small of her back, and along her rib cage, moving slowly and sensually.

4 Pucker your lips and give a wet suck to her nipples, while adding a little tongue around her areola. Place a ravishing kiss on her neck and nibble her ears.

5 Slide your lips over her abdomen and tongue her navel. Raise and spread her legs, giving her a very wet and sloppy kiss on her perineum and entire vulva.

6 Tongue fuck her vagina with a firm tongue. Slurp your way to her clit, where you wrap your lips around her clit as you suckle and tongue her to orgasm.

7 Embrace her. Kiss her forehead and eyes with caring and sensitivity.

THE SEXPERT SAYS

Think of kissing as a medium for what you want to communicate. For better structure, imagine a kissing sandwich, where you kiss at the beginning, middle, and end, making intention the heart of your kisses.

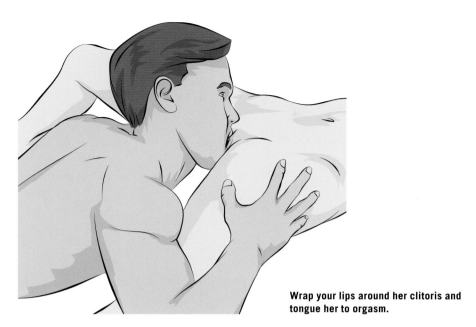

Wrap your lips around her clitoris and tongue her to orgasm.

RELATED MOVES

★ Place a barrier (condom, dental dam, plastic wrap) over her anus and rim her, also known as kissing her ass. If she doesn't like anal sex, she might still like this.

★ Kissing can also be an effective tool for helping you last longer. Pause intercourse when you are in high arousal, well before the point of no return, and kiss her (anywhere) to take attention off you and on to her. Resume and repeat.

♀ WHY IT WORKS FOR HER

★ Did I mention that women love kissing? Women equate kissing with sexual satisfaction, which means the more kissing, the more satisfied they are with the sex.

★ Like you, women also savor anticipation. All this attention is going to have her peaking in high arousal way before you put your mouth on her clit.

♂ WHY IT WORKS FOR HIM

★ The saying "The tongue is more powerful than the sword" could not be truer in this instance. Many women need oral sex in order to climax. You have the sword.

★ This move will give you great oral sex skills and techniques in mastering the art of seduction.

★ The position also allows you to engage all of your senses at once: seeing her, feeling her, tasting her, hearing her, and smelling her, which all contribute to intensifying your orgasm.

|||||||||||||||||||||||||||||||||||||||||||||||||||||||||||||||||||||||||||||||||||||||||||||||||||||||||||

SEX FACT

Kissing each day will keep the dentist away and give you fresh breath. Kissing encourages saliva to wash food from the teeth and lowers the level of the acid that causes decay, preventing plaque buildup. (Still, brush your teeth and carry mints.)

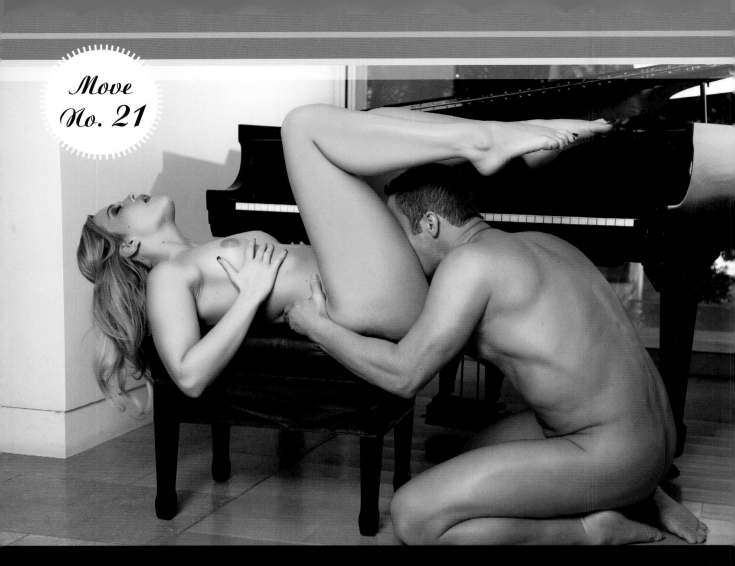

OH MY GODDESS

Much like a man becoming a knight must kneel before the queen who bestows his knighthood, this scenario will have you prove your worthiness with your tongue. Of all the men in the kingdom, you are the chosen one who is begging for a chance with her. You are the one lucky enough to worship her, lucky enough to be licking her royal clit, and lucky enough to show your devotion to her. Leave your ego at the door and watch your goddess in the glow of being worshiped.

Being worshiped is a common female fantasy, and here's a chance to enjoy making your goddess's dreams come true. If you've never paid homage to her vulva, pay particular close attention to this move, do it regularly, and watch her glow.

The Move: Oh My Goddess

THE PREPARATIONS

★ Get into the space of sincere appreciation for your goddess. If you can't come up with something off the top of your head, you are not in the spirit of appreciating your goddess. Pick up a pen and start listing what you love/lust about her, and how she makes your world a brighter place.

★ Clean the space, light candles, and play some relaxing music.

★ Decorate her goddess chair. It's okay if it doesn't look perfect. She will get the thought and the signal that this is something special. Place a pretty piece of fabric over an ordinary chair and place a small pillow against the back. The pillow is obviously to show that you care about her comfort, but also to push her forward a bit so she can sit with her vulva hanging over the chair edge. The fabric can be a throw blanket, silk scarf, sarong, or pretty sheet.

★ To learn more about what she likes orally, blindfold her or ask her to close her eyes, then ask her to rate the following oral techniques from 1 to 5:

- Feathers: Make ever-so-light brushes of the tongue across the clit.
- Painting the Walls: Make large, flat strokes on the inner walls of the labia.
- Nibbles: Cover your teeth with your lips and give her little nibbles. Does she prefer fast and furious or slow and sensual?
- The Vibrator: Press your lips against her clit and hum to vibrate them.
- Rimming: Lick her ass. Spread her butt cheeks and run your tongue over the pucker of her anus. For sanitary reasons, I recommend placing a barrier, such as a dental dam or piece of plastic wrap, over the area.
- Flickering: Flicker your tongue across her clit.
- Upper Lip Press: Press the upper lip against the commissure for pressure and move your head back and forth as if rubbing your mouth.
- Suck and Twirl: Suck and add the twirling of your tongue over the clitoris.
- Tongue Fuck: Insert your tongue into her vagina.
- Pressure: Add pressure with a firm tongue.
- Location: Where does she like to be stimulated: U-spot, clitoral glans, commissure, labia?

SEX FACT

Reportedly, the T'ang Dynasty empress Wu Hu required all visiting dignitaries to perform oral sex on her. (True or not, it's a nice thought!)

- Penetration: Does she like a finger insertion? If so, how many fingers and how much depth does she like?
- Suction: Wrap your lips around the base of her clit and suck. If she likes suction, find out how much.
- Patterns: Does she like you to do circles or figure eights, or tongue the alphabet?

★ You don't need pen and paper for this exercise, but take note of the 4s and 5s, but maybe more important is how she liked it overall. Keep practicing. This exercise is commonly used for pre-orgasmic women or women who can't climax with oral sex. It is also perfect for longtime couples to spice up their sex life because now you have a shared language and understanding of what she likes.

THE LEAD-IN

Send flowers to your goddess along with the list of all the things you appreciate about her. Add a p.s.: "My Excellency, your wish is my command. Be ready to receive."

When she walks in the door, look in her eyes, get down on your knees, and tell her what you love about her. Yeah, sure, you sent it in the letter, but she wants to hear you say it, too.

THE FOREPLAY

① Still kneeling, begin to kiss her feet. Help her take off her shoes and begin to kiss, lick, and suck each of her toes. Slowly kiss your way up her calves, pausing at the back of the knees for a little suction and twirl of the tongue. She will recognize the suction and tongue move from oral sex and begin to build up the anticipation as you get closer and closer to her royal jewels.

② Close your eyes and move your way up to her inner thighs. Really get into the moment. Feel your lips against her soft skin, smell her musk, feel her warmth, and taste her essence. Be so in the moment that you are feeling your cock getting hard with just a kiss; be so in the moment that you could feel her inner thighs receiving the kiss and kissing you back. Being in the moment is the trademark of a great lover. Being in the moment is also used as a practice to manage early ejaculation.

|||||||||||||||||||||||||||||||||||||||||||||||||||||||||||||||||||||||||||||||||||||||||||||||||||||||||||||||||||||||||

SEX FACT

"When a man sits with a pretty girl for an hour, it seems like a minute . . . That's relativity."

—Albert Einstein

3. Plead with her to let you lick her heaven and earth, her pussy. Say, "Please, please, please. I want to smell and taste you."

4. If she gets the game and refuses, she wants more begging. Give it to her and lay it on thick.

5. If she still resists, start smaller, settle for a lick of her nipple, then her ass, until she gives in and lets you lick her pussy. Look up at her and ever so gently glide your tongue up her thighs, giving her a seductive tease. Remember that emotional and psychological stimulation is an important part of seduction and sex.

6. While she is still standing and you are on your knees, put your hands on her rear and your face in her pussy. Move your nose over her clit and in between her folds. Let her see you inhaling the unique scent of her pussy. Use your tongue to trace her labia and the base of her clitoris with a soft, slow movement so she can feel every sensation.

7. Use a flat tongue and cover the inside of her labia so she can feel the texture and firmness of your tongue. Run the same firm tongue up and down the commissure, avoiding the clitoral glans.

8. Put saliva on your finger and smooth it over the pucker of her asshole.

9. Start circling her clitoris with your tongue as if circling your prey. Enjoy the seductive and teasing dance, knowing that you will get to her clit eventually, but until then both of you are enjoying the anticipation.

10. When she starts to squirm and get weak in the knees, take her to the royal throne you have prepared.

||||||||||||||||||||||||||||||||||||||||||||||||||||||||||||||||||||||||||||||||||||||||||||||||||||||||||||||||||

SEX FACT

Touch decreases stress and releases "feel good" hormones such as oxytocin, nature's bonding agent. The release in hormones increases sexual responsiveness and sensitivity.

★ The Main Act

1 Sit her in her goddess chair, get down on your knees, and spread her legs.

2 Tell her that you are going to be her servant of desire, doing whatever she asks, but you will need directions to her kingdom. Tell her that you want her to command how you lick her vulva as if you were her personal sex toy. You know that there isn't one that can even come close to the sensations your mouth can provide. You prepared yourselves with the earlier exercise, and now she can tell you what she wants.

3 Wait there for a moment with your face in her royal crotch, letting her feel your breath and giving ever-so-soft touches of your tongue. Your touch is so soft that it tickles.

4 Switch gears only when she gives you a command to do something else. Changing directions is fine, but nothing major.

5 The other move that is okay to do without her specific instructions is putting pressure on the commissure with your upper lip. The commissure is a chord of nerve fibers that feeds the entire clitoris. Pressure here feels good without overstimulating the clitoris, making it a staple move.

6 While you are waiting, rub your free hand over her nipples and slipping her nipples between your fingers. Nipple stimulation can help bring some women over the top.

7 If either of you is getting uncomfortable, it may be time for an adjustment. She can rest her foot/feet on your shoulders or chest. This will significantly open her up and give you better access.

8 Follow her lead, doing what she likes when she likes it: sucking, flicking, licking, and twirling, until she screams, "Oh my goddess!" During resolution, look up at her and remind her of all the things you cherish about her sexually.

9 After she's climaxed, you can give her another orgasm orally or do the related move. After orgasm, women are still highly orgasmic and don't need to necessarily go through the entire sexual response cycle for another O.

THE SEXPERT SAYS

It's one thing to have sex with your partner and another to be wanted by your partner. Give your partner the opportunity to *want* and *be wanted* with seductive scenarios like this one. A large part of arousal is believing that your partner sincerely wants you.

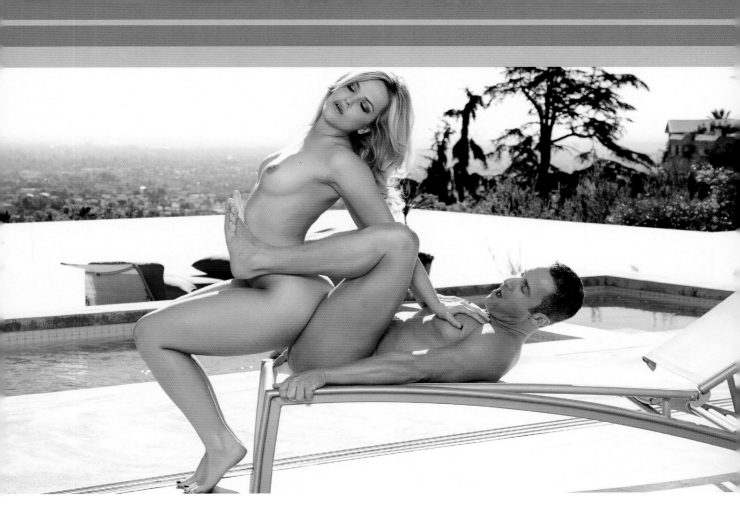

RELATED MOVES

★ If you want to keep the same theme, but have intercourse, you be the chair. To get into this position, lie on your back, spread your legs, and hold your knees to your shoulders, forming a sort of a throne. She sits on the back of your thighs and mounts you. (See above.)

♀ WHY IT WORKS FOR HER

★ She gives it up for you readily and often, but that doesn't mean she doesn't want to be wanted, begged and pleaded with for her magic vulva from time to time. It's a fact that women need more foreplay than men do; remember, sex starts in the brain.

♂ WHY IT WORKS FOR HIM

★ If you don't love giving her oral sex, Oh My Goddess may change your mind. You will never forget seeing her in the glow of being worshiped. This position will help you give your oral gift with great intention.

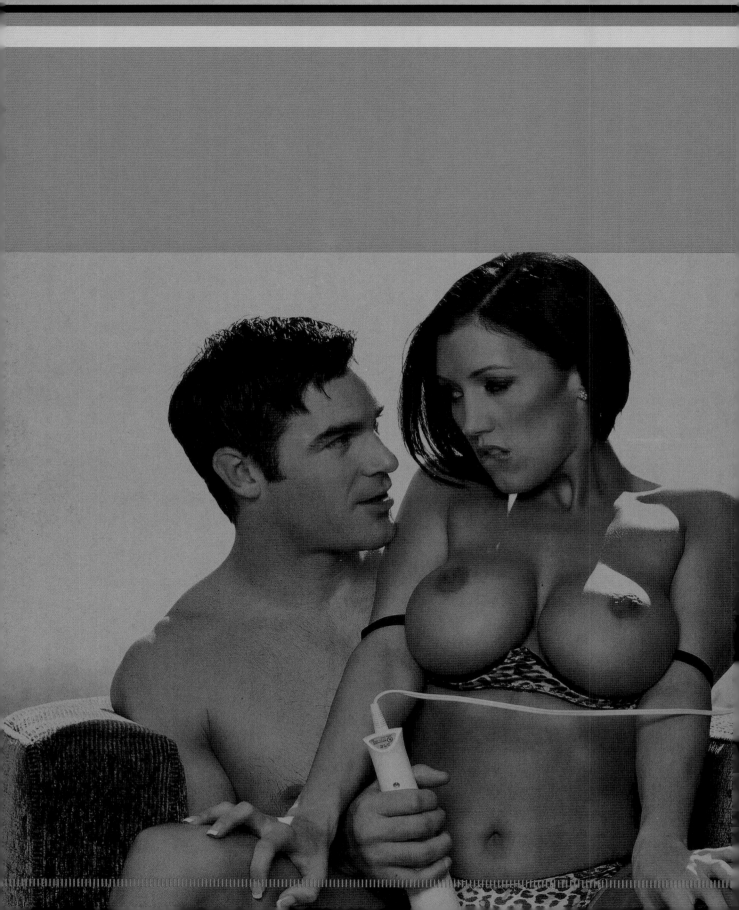

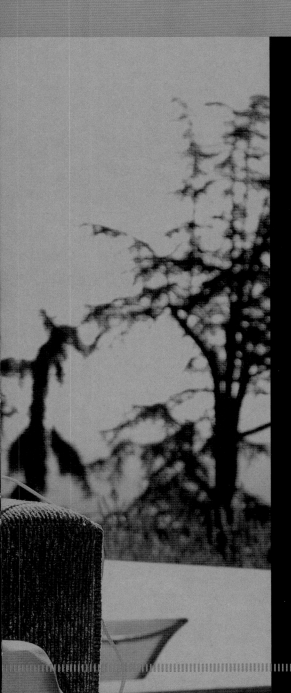

Hand Jobs

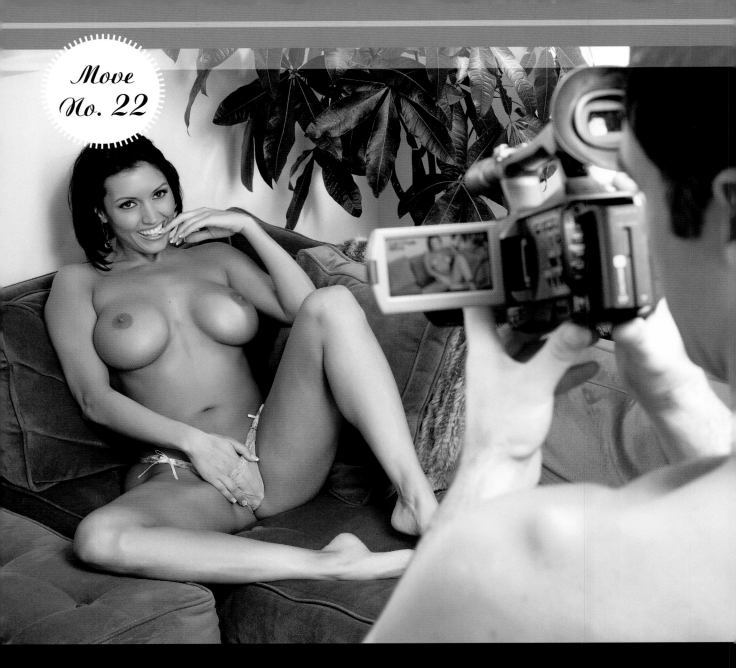

★ SEX 101

Lights. Camera. Action. Turn ordinary masturbation into a red-hot, potentially life-changing experience for both of you by making your own sex flicks. In this move, you will uncover the secrets that make her soar and become the best lover each of you has ever had.

The Move: Sex 101

THE PREPARATIONS

★ You want to gather information about your lover so you can create the set for your movie. Choose a good time for the interview, perhaps over wine and a great meal or after lovemaking. Make it playful and fun, asking questions such as, What do you do to get into the mood (music, candles, warm bath)? Where do you masturbate? Do you have certain thoughts or fantasies that get you hot? What position do you masturbate in? What parts of your body do you stimulate? If you were to make a porno film, what would your porn name be? Tell her that you think it would be fun to make a porno film with her and then watch it together.

★ Once you've gathered this great information, set up a masturbation station and pull together the things that help her get into the mood, blindfolds, anything else she might use, and something new that she has never used before, such as a new toy or a female enhancement gel (this can make the clitoris more sensitive and add new sensations to the usual masturbation session).

★ If it's cool, turn up the heat. Eventually, things will get hot, but you want her to be comfortable.

★ Set up a camcorder and tripod. Practice turning it on and zooming in and out.

★ Dim the lights, but no darkness. You want to be able to see this show.

THE LEAD-IN

Go bold and send her a text that says, "Dinner and a porno tonight starring you and me. Wear your favorite sexy outfit. See you at 7:00. I made reservations at your favorite restaurant."

Set up the masturbation station.

THE FOREPLAY

① Send her a text that day calling her by her porno name; have fun and tease her with naughty thoughts. Let your mind go wild thinking about her masturbating.

② Be prepared for a night of foreplay (that is, if you want a mind-blowing porno!). On your way to the restaurant, put your hand on her leg, look at her, and smile like you know a secret, because you do. Run your fingers up and down her legs and sneak kisses during red lights. Don't leave the light until someone honks.

③ When you arrive at the restaurant, treat her like the lady she is: take her coat, pull out her chair, and so on (remember, she's not a real porn star!). After you order, tell her about how you can't get her out of your mind and how the visions of her bringing herself to orgasm creeps in during business meetings and makes you do mindless things. Then kiss her like a helpless romantic.

4. During dinner, rub her legs, play footsies, and ask her to describe her fantasies. Angle yourself for a peek of her breasts or inner thigh.

5. Keep up the play. If you feel awkward and don't know what to say, kiss her, massage her, and tell her everything that makes her beautiful. Make a toast to her beauty. Feed her food in a loving way. Make sure she has a glass of wine (or two!) to help her relax.

6. When you get her back to the house, take her to the masturbation station that you have set up and show her everything that she loves to play with as well as the "something new." You may forget her birthday, but the fact that you remembered what she loves to masturbate with will please her to no end.

7. Remind her that you are going to delete the film when you're done, because this will help her relax in front of the camera. Turn on the camera and ask her to get undressed.

8. Encourage her as she disrobes in front of you. Remind her what parts turn you on (or the parts of her that you love best). Feeling aroused yet? Tell her how she turns you on.

9. Once she's naked, put a little female enhancement gel on your finger and place it on her clitoris. Kiss whatever she is opening up and exposing to you: her neck, her breasts, her ears. Kiss it all.

10. Check the camera and assure her that she looks great. Women are always concerned about how they look on camera, so let the excitement roar and tell her how much the camera loves her.

||||||||||||||||||||||||||||||||||||||||||||||||||||||||||||||||||||||||||||||||||||||||||||||||||||||||||||

SEX FACT

People keep their same masturbation patterns throughout their life, unless they consciously choose to change them. Often the same is true for sex with a partner: it's the same unless they choose to change it.

||||||||||||||||||||||||||||||||||||||||||||||||||||||||||||||||||||||||||||||||||||||||||||||||||||||||||||

THE SEXPERT SAYS

This scenario is not just smoking hot, but it's also an amazing way to learn about your own and each other's sexuality, making you both the best lovers you can be. It's a great way to create shared, sexy experiences that you will never forget. I dare you to make a series.

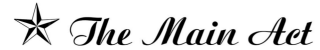 # The Main Act

1 Take off your clothes and get into your masturbation position while still in the camera's view. Put on the blindfolds and stroke, touch, and fantasize as you would during masturbation. (If it turns you on, talk to each other about what you're doing, how you're touching yourself, and what it feels like; alternatively, save this conversation for when you watch the movie together.)

2 Excited to see the movie? Pop the popcorn, pour the drinks, and watch the movie. As you watch, describe what you are doing through the entire sexual response cycle. Tell each other about your thoughts and strokes during early arousal, increased arousal, and before orgasm to orgasm and resolution.

3 Describe pressure, pace, rhythm, and direction in details: "I am loosely gripping my cock with my right hand and occasionally rubbing my fingers over the head. Now, with my other hand, I am playing with my balls and pulling them down a little bit during increased arousal because it helps me last longer. And right here, I am thinking about putting my cock in your ass. Look—that thought almost put me over the top. You have a great ass. I had to pause. I am starting back up again with the same stroke and pinching my nipples. I love to have my nipples played with."

4 Ask if you can show her the stroke. Reach for her hand and show her the pressure, pace, and rhythm of your motions.

5 Now, it's her turn. Give her your hand and ask her to show you the stroke that takes her to infinity and beyond.

6 Don't forget to delete the film when you're done!

7 She will never forget the porno you made together. When things get a little predictable, park the camcorder in front of the bed for her to see. She'll get the hint.

RELATED MOVES

★ You can do this one by one, or side by side without the blindfolds. You can also do this move long distance over the phone or with Skype if someone goes on a trip.

♀ WHY IT WORKS FOR HER

★ You will know what she likes and exactly how to touch her. This is a great exercise if she is orgasmically challenged with a partner.

♂ WHY IT WORKS FOR HIM

★ This one move alone can save you hours of time and put you on the top of your game right away.

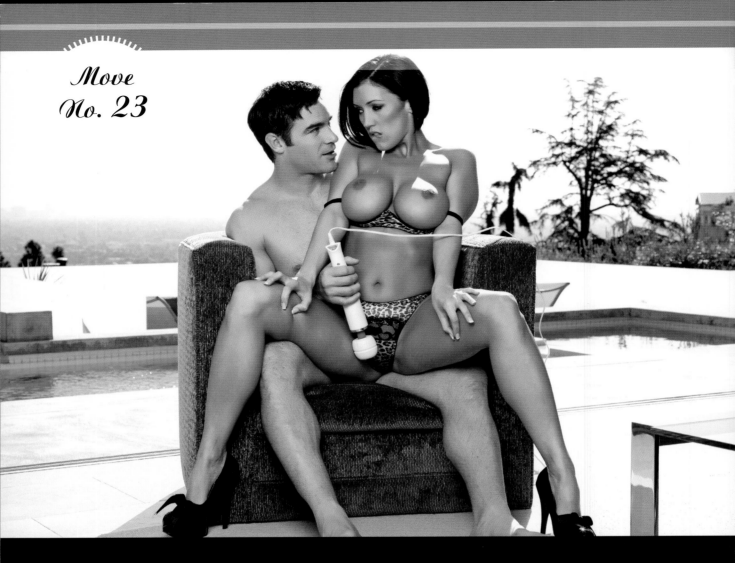

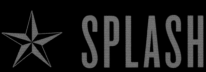 # SPLASH

Female ejaculation can be very empowering for your girl. At the very least, it can be a fun, shared sex adventure (is there a better kind?). You can use this scenario to learn the process and coach her through it with a few simple techniques.

When a woman is aroused, the Skene's glands, or paraurethral glands, produce an alkaline liquid. These glands are similar to the male prostate gland, and the alkaline liquid is similar to seminal fluid. Female ejaculation can range from a few drops to several tablespoons and can be brought on with clitoral or vaginal stimulation.

The Move: Splash

THE PREPARATIONS

★ Lay down a towel to eliminate any concern about "mess." Do this regularly, starting with the first time your lover attempts female ejaculation, so there is assurance that any night can be a female ejaculation night.

★ Make sure she knows she is safe to go with the feeling of needing to pee. Even if she did make a mess it would be okay. This assurance is very important to the process.

★ Purchase *The Art of Female Ejaculation* DVD by Lisa Lawless and a high-speed vibrator such as the Hitachi Magic Wand. Wrap the vibrator.

★ It's likely that she won't ejaculate on the first try. If she's nervous, one option is to have her practice on her own during masturbation with the Hitachi Magic Wand and then come together for more practice sessions. Do it all in the spirit of fun play.

THE LEAD-IN

Tell her you want to try female ejaculation for fun. Establish a "no pressure" approach by letting her know that it would be fun to "try." This will show her that you enjoy the journey and are not just concerned about the end result. Women get performance anxiety, too.

When you get a "yes," hand her the present, insert the DVD, and click play.

THE FOREPLAY

① Watch the DVD together. If you are willing to deal with the interruptions of streaming video, you can also view it at www.xhamster.com for free.

② Go slow and build a psychologically and physically arousing time for your lover. Spend time sucking on her nipples. Let her see you flicking a pointed tongue over her nipples, then trace them using a circular motion. Gently suck on them, increasing the pressure while adding stimulation with your tongue.

||||||||||||||||||||||||||||||||||||||||||||||||||||||||||||||||||||||||||||||||||||||||||||||||||||||||||||||||||||||||

SEX FACT

Some women ejaculate a little, others a lot, and the rest somewhere in between. It may be inconsistent, which means that she may emit fluid some days and not others. Lastly, it may not be as sensational an experience or feeling as she expected. This is just for fun, so if she is not interested or enjoying the process, don't push it. An experience that is "empowering" to some may just be a fun exercise to others. No expectations.

★ The Main Act

1. The most common ways to bring about female ejaculation are through vaginal stimulation (usually G-spot), clitoral stimulation, or both. The most important thing to remember is the process. Once she nails the process and the new feelings that accompany it, you will both be able to experiment with different forms.

2. If you are trying this for the first time, I recommend the vibrator and clitoral stimulation over the vibrator with G-spot stimulation. The latter is a lot of stimulation and it seems to be less effective, especially when learning the process is the most important part.

3. There are two methods for bringing on female ejaculation:

   Vaginal G-Spot Stimulation for Female Ejaculation: Have her lie on her back on the bed with her legs bent and her rear close to the edge while you kneel on the floor. Insert a clean, lubricated finger or G-spot stimulator 2 to 3 inches (5 to 7.5 cm) inside the vagina along the upper part of the vaginal wall (tummy side), pressing it toward the pelvis in a "come here" motion. The G-spot will feel spongy when at rest and firm when aroused. Start out slow, then increase the pressure and possibly the rate of movement. Ask her what she needs. Watch her body and listen for feedback. Using lube, saliva, or the lubrication from her vagina, begin gently rubbing her clitoris with the fingers of your other hand. Even though you are focusing on a G-spot orgasm, give her some clitoral stimulation; some women can't climax without it.

   Clitoral Stimulation for Female Ejaculation: Using a finger is more sensual and a different sensation, but if you are going to go with vibrating clitoral stimulation, I suggest using a high-powered vibrator, such as the Hitachi Magic Wand. The vibrator is great because it may empower her to practice on her own.

4. Continue to keep her in high arousal. Remind her to relax and breathe and that she can squirt over into the next room and you would be thrilled.

5. If she is inclined, have her masturbate and tell you what she is doing. If she is not, take her on an experience, hold the vibrator, and share a visualization of what she might expect. Put your hand on her abdomen and say, "Close your eyes and enjoy. Relax and breathe. Take your awareness to the sensations. Notice the possible tingly, cool, or warm feelings. Notice your Skene's glands filling with fluid."

6. When she begins to have contractions, have her breathe and relax through them; this in itself will build the tension, ultimately creating a more intense orgasm.

7. Tell her, "It's going to feel like you need to pee, but it's not urine, so go ahead and tell yourself it is okay and let go. The orgasm feels differently than pee. It feels electrifying." Embracing the need to "pee" is probably the biggest barrier, but once she passes this the process gets easier and easier.

8. Love, kiss, and celebrate her, regardless of whether she ejaculates or not. Talk about it and find out how the process felt for her.

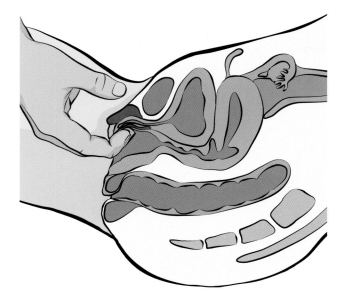

Insert your finger in a couple inches into her vagina along the upper part of the vaginal wall and press it torward the pelvis as if you are beckoning "come here."

RELATED MOVES

★ She can ejaculate during intercourse, too. Once you determine where she needs stimulation in order to ejaculate, you can choose the appropriate position.

♀ WHY IT WORKS FOR HER

★ She will love the newfound control, power, and intimacy with her own body.

★ In addition, many women who ejaculate report that their orgasms are more intense. Others aren't sure what the big deal is.

♂ WHY IT WORKS FOR HIM

★ Men who are part of a woman's ejaculation report feeling a stronger connection with her from the shared experience.

★ Female ejaculation gives you more feedback. With this new feedback comes more familiarity with her sexual response cycle and control over her orgasms.

THE SEXPERT SAYS

Part of the psychological arousal with this scenario involves the feeling of trust, safety, and acceptance to let go and enjoy a probably unfamiliar bodily response. Talk about the process with her. What was it like? Listen, learn, and enjoy.

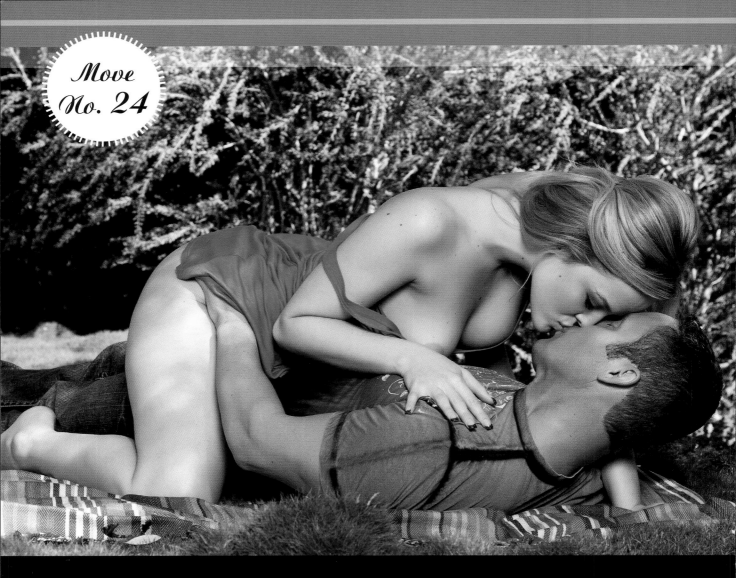

SUMMER CONCERT

It will be the best concert she has ever seen no matter who is playing. Join the band as you hit all the high and low notes with your own sonata. You will single-handedly learn how to digitally delight her under the picnic blanket and give her a world-class orgasm while never looking under the blanket. Now that's a pro!

Summer will come and go and the years will pass, but she will never forget the orgasm you gave her under the blanket.

The Move: Summer Concert

THE PREPARATIONS

★ Find a summer concert in your area that goes until the evening. Stay away from the Hannah Montana types of concerts that attract underage youth.

★ Clip your fingernails and pack the warming lube and some hand wipes for comfortable digital play. Bring along several blankets.

★ Invite her to the concert and tell her you would love to see her in a long skirt (but no panties).

★ Pack a picnic basket of her favorite most indulgent picnic foods and don't forget the chocolate. If you don't know her favorite foods, ask. Thoughtfulness will always take you far.

THE LEAD-IN

Pull out the delicious food and drink you've packed in the basket and show her the warming lube. When she asks what it is for, connect your eyes, touch her face, and just before you kiss her, whisper that she is part of the chorus tonight. Bring a hand down from her face, brush it against her nipple, and rest it on her inner thigh.

Kiss her by softly brushing your lips against hers, moving your head back and forth, feeling her warm breath and smiling at her with your eyes. Gently press your lips so you can go in for a deeper kiss. Close your eyes and let the sun relax you. Feel her energy and yours meeting at the lips. Wow! That's hot. Now turn up the tease with the slide in of your tongue, then pull it out before engaging in serious tongue tango. When you end the kiss, *slowly* pull back so you can watch each other's bliss.

THE FOREPLAY

① Hand-feed her the food items from the picnic basket one by one in courses, taking time to play with the food in a sensual way.

② Roll a juicy ripe strawberry over her lips, along her jaw, and down her neck, before allowing her to take a bite. Hold a piece of chocolate in your mouth just long enough for it to melt a bit, and then lean in and kiss her, using your tongue to push the chocolate into her mouth.

③ Turn an ordinary picnic into a "wow" picnic with the best spice of all, sexiness. Think of the classic movie *Like Water for Chocolate*, and set the intention for *hot*.

④ Take a small bite of a food, such as a juicy grape. Hold it up so she can see and slowly bring it to her mouth. Do a few Kegels between each bite. Kegels bring blood flow and energy to your genitals and are great to do when you want to turn on the heat. Feed her a bite of food and this time trail her lips with it. Kegels. With the next bite, follow up the trail with a simple kiss. Kegels. For the next bite, act as if you are going to feed her, then drop a little on her neck and suck it off.

⑤ Point out why the night is so special: "What a great night. I'm so lucky. Perfect weather, great music, and an amazing woman."

⑥ Be attentive to her needs. Try to anticipate and offer what she might need. Water? Wine? Shoulder rub?

⑦ Cuddle and snuggle her. Lay your head in her lap.

⑧ Get her comfortable. Have her put her legs out in front of her and her hands behind her back. Lie between her legs on your side with your upper body propped up with your arm and your head on her belly; feel your head rise and fall with every breath, letting it relax and ground you.

⑨ Occasionally, turn your head and press your lips against her inner thighs or abdomen and hum to the song; this will send vibrations up her spine. Cover your teeth with your lips, take a bite of her clothed flesh, and hum.

★ The Main Act

1 When the sun sets, cover her legs and lap with the blanket so it looks to everyone else that it is a pillow for your head or you are trying to keep warm.

2 Slip your hand under the blanket. Glide a finger into her vagina, reaching back toward her cervix and stopping at the anterior fornix erogenous (AFE) zone for some of her own lubrication. Alternatively, you can always discretely use bottled lube.

3 On your way down from the AFE zone continue to glide your fingers down the front wall of the vagina and rub her G-spot.

4 Spread the lubrication between her labia and along the base of her clitoral shaft. Using your thumb and index finger, apply light pinching pressure while giving long strokes up and down her clit as if you were stroking your cock. After about four long strokes, feather a finger over the "head" of her clit.

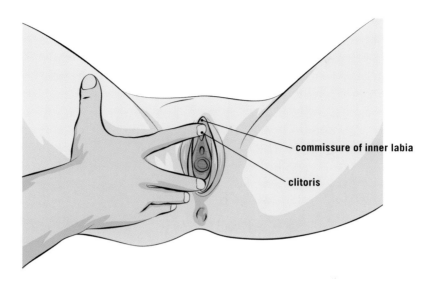

commissure of inner labia

clitoris

SEX FACT

David Gibson at the Sound and Consciousness Institute in San Francisco reports that if you want to bring love into the bedroom, look for music that has a slow tempo to breathe to. Slow tempos resonate love, while fast tempos activate and excite.

5 Once you have given her clit a fair introduction, strum it. Place your middle or ring finger on her commissure for pressure and mild rubbing while you use your index finger, the one with the most dexterity, to move across and up and down the clit.

6 Switch the pattern of your index finger to a circle. Keep one finger rubbing the commissure. Imagine the clitorial shaft is the downhill mountain and the clitoral glans is the cliff. When you get to the clitoral cliff, occasionally tap and then move back up the mountain for more pressure.

7 Play her like chords: stroke the clitoris with tempo and rhythm, all in time with the music.

8 More importantly, pay close attention to her own beat and rhythm. With your head on her belly, you can hear her breathe and feel her contractions.

9 When she is in high arousal, press your non-strumming hand firmly just above her pubic bone to externally stimulate her G-spot. She will likely respond to the pressure by pushing out and contracting her muscles, bringing more blood flow to the genitals and facilitating the orgasmic process.

10 Place the thumb of your strumming hand on her commissure and massage the clit up and down. Insert the index and pointer fingers of your strumming hand into her vagina and press on her G-spot, now adding internal pressure.

11 Bring her all the way to the end, slowing down and decreasing pressure on the clit with each contraction as she orgasms.

12 Sit up and move behind her. Cover her with your arms and enjoy the concert. Whisper in her ear what you loved about sharing that with her.

13 If the band is selling a CD, buy one and play it during your indoor, midwinter picnic.

|||||||||||||||||||||||||||||||||||||||||||||||||||||||||||||||||||||||||||||||||||||||||||||||||||||||||||||||||||

SEX FACT

Chocolate contains phenylethylamine, the same chemical responsible for the high of sexual attraction and being in love.

RELATED MOVES

★ Sitting behind her, reach in and rub her clit to orgasm. Unless you have long arms, you won't get as good penetration with this move, but you will get to sing in her ear. Use your other hand to gently pinch her nipple as you stimulate her clit.

♀ WHY IT WORKS FOR HER

★ Most women need an emotional connection to make sex more enjoyable, and a romantic and relaxed setting such as an outdoor concert provides that. She will feel more in sync with you as you bring her to climax.

★ Being fingered is a totally amazing experience if the giver is skilled (and you are!). Add the thrill of having an orgasm in public and she may be asking for an encore performance.

♂ WHY IT WORKS FOR HIM

★ Sexual interactions in a public setting are always exciting and dangerous. Most men thrive on this and it will drive you wild even as you drive her wild.

★ Your other senses will be awakened without relying on your sight for sexual feedback. All this sharpens your skills as a lover.

THE SEXPERT SAYS

Orgasm is much, much more than just a physiological response. Think about engaging her on all levels: physical, emotional, spiritual, and psychological. Our bodies are more responsive to pleasure when we feel loved and appreciated.

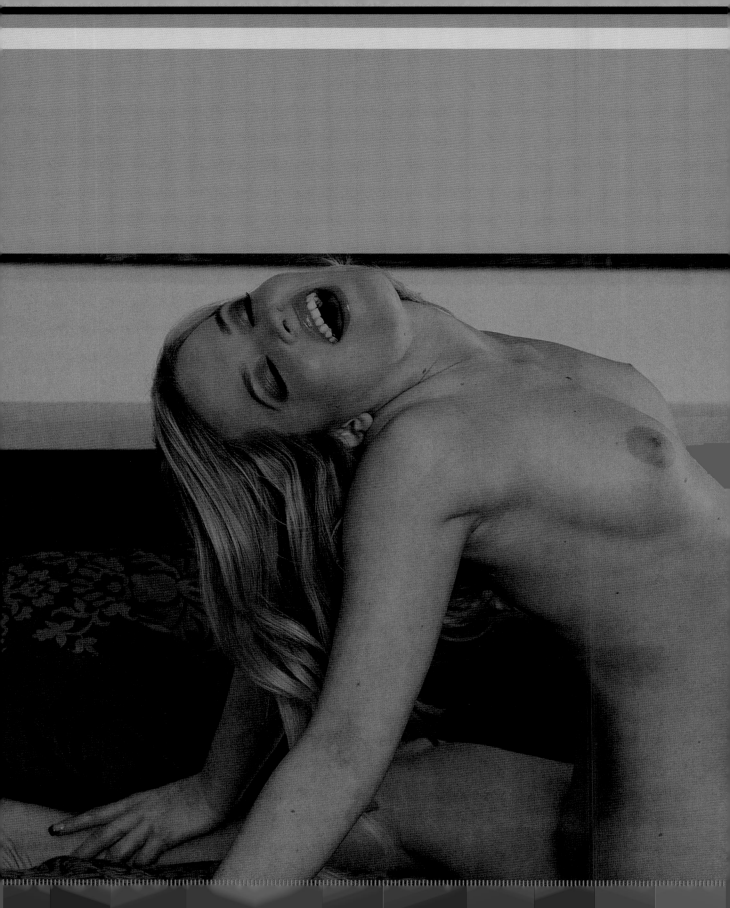

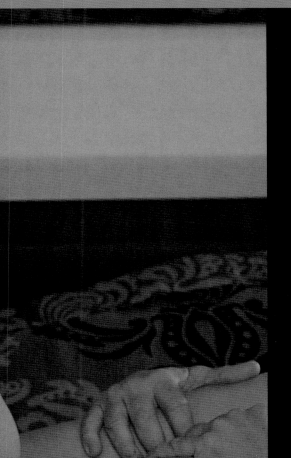

Moregasms

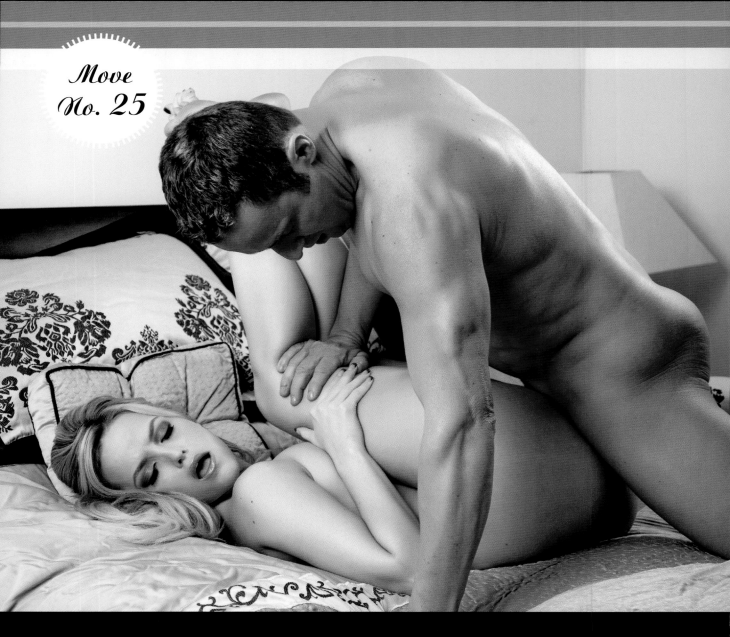

 # BLUE PUSSY

Women have their own version of blue balls; it's called blue pussy. This is not a sad puss—quite the contrary. We are talking about a highly aroused, anticipatory pussy that eventually becomes a very satisfied pussy. The heavy foreplay here will have her spreading her legs, craving your cock for deep penetration, and coming back for more.

The Move: Blue Pussy

THE PREPARATIONS

★ Think back to the images of her masturbating in the Sex 101 scenario. What did she do to bring herself to high arousal? Did she play music? If yes, have that music ready. Music can be an anchor, which can help us get to our state of arousal in a moment. Baseball players kick the dirt before they throw a pitch so they can get into the right space for playing ball. Now, you play music to help put her in the right place for orgasm. You are masterful.

★ If you are not already familiar with the magic of the cervix, get acquainted. Slide her down to the edge of the bed with her knees bent. Visualize her anatomy so you know what you are looking for. The narrow end of the uterus that connects it with the top of the vagina is the cervix. It feels hard to the touch and expands with arousal and orgasm. The fornices have been described as a ringlike structure that encircles the cervix, with the texture similar to that of the back of a Frisbee.

★ Press down with one finger on her vagina opening, slowly inserting a finger. Press on the G-spot as you enter. Move farther up the vaginal canal and press on the cervix—feel its shape and texture with the pad of your finger.

★ Find the posterior fornix by sliding your finger up the front vaginal wall, bypassing the G-spot, until you feel firmness (the cervix). Now, slide your finger down a wee bit until you feel a small gap between the cervix and the vaginal wall. This is the posterior fornix. Gently press there, then rotate your finger.

THE LEAD-IN

Give her a copy of my book, *Spectacular Sex Moves He'll Never Forget*. Write a note that says, "I am reading *Spectacular Sex Moves She'll Never Forget*. Let's choose one chapter each and do it tonight."

Place the note inside the book so it is hanging out and clearly visible. Wrap the sexy book and leave it for her to open before she leaves the house. This could be a great way to suggest many more sexcapades in the future.

Send her a text that says, "Tonight, I want you to feel your arousal. I want you to feel the pleasure but delay orgasm. You must resist coming."

THE FOREPLAY

1. When she walks in the door, walk her to the wall, get really close as if you are going to kiss her lips, but don't. Instead, look her in the eye and rub a finger over her nipple and have her tell you about her day.

2. Move her hair aside and blow warm breath in her ears. Open her shirt and inch your fingers into her bra. Rub your pelvis against hers so she can feel the hardness of your cock. Open her blouse and tease your tongue around the areolas of her breasts. Twirl a wet tongue on the nipples and blow.

3. Place her hands behind her back and tell her to spread her legs. Tell her the rule of the game is resist. Keep her in the standing position until she is begging you to fuck her.

4. Get down on your knees and breathe more warm breath on her mons. Insert your tongue between her labia so lightly that she is not sure if you are tickling her or licking her. You are lickling.

5. Turn her around, spread her cheeks, and kiss her ass. Gently spank her bare bottom so the entire 15,000-nerve network in her pelvis region gets a vibration. Ever so lightly, lickle the letter "T" on her clit. Do the whole alphabet in lickles, stopping every five letters for a spank. Resume.

6. When you see her in high arousal, gently run your fingernails over her abdomen and pubic hairs.

8. Reach up and twirl her nipples from time to time. There is no hurry. Be ruthless and pull out whatever technique you learned from the masturbation movie.

9. Keep going until you hear the sweet words, "Fuck me."

||||||||||||||||||||||||||||||||||||||||||||||||||||||||||||||||||||||||||||||||||||||||||||||||||||||||||||||||||||||

SEX FACT

When a female rhinoceros is feeling in the mood, she will ram her potential lover with her horn. Hence, the word *horny*.

||||||||||||||||||||||||||||||||||||||||||||||||||||||||||||||||||||||||||||||||||||||||||||||||||||||||||||||||||||||

THE SEXPERT SAYS

It's great to know techniques, positions, and moves, but our largest sex organ is our brain. If you learn how to arouse, you can bring her to climax in minutes, again and again.

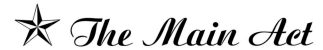

★ The Main Act

1 Take her to the bed, lay her on her back, spread her legs, and hold her knees to her chest so her rear is lifted.

2 Get on your knees and lean over her so you are several inches above her. Insert your cock slowly. When you get to the end of the vagina, press your pelvis so she gets it deep. Try focusing the thrusting energy in your hips, rather than your whole body, so she gets all your concentrated efforts.

3 This is not the traditional fucking with the full-on thrusts and removal and insertion of your penis; this is more about giving her pleasure, like you did in the Clitty Cat. But this time, you are doing all that and going for more depth and pressure on the cervix zone that comes with the knees-to-chest position. Remember to be conscious of having contact with her clit.

4 Move your pelvis back and forth as if you are massaging her with your cock. Whisper in her ear and talk about how she is a dirty girl who likes to get fucked and who needs to get fucked. Each time you say the word *fucked*, give it to her a little deeper, a little harder, until her blue pussy is a happy pussy.

RELATED MOVES

★ Access the AFE zone via the anus and the vagina. Slowly insert a finger in her vagina until you feel the cervix, or the back wall. Push the finger toward her rear and upward. Slowly insert another well-lubed finger into her anus, pointing toward the front of her body. Gently press. The finger in the anus not only massages the AFE, but it also narrows the vaginal cavity, allowing for more stimulation along the vaginal walls.

♀ WHY IT WORKS FOR HER

★ She will be amazed at how quickly she becomes aroused and lubricated with all the foreplay and stimulation to the clitoris and cervix zone.

♂ WHY IT WORKS FOR HIM

★ You will love going deep inside her, giving her a potentially major release. Cervical spot orgasms have been known to bring about an emotional and physical release. If she does have a release, simply holding her, giving her eye contact, opening your heart, and listening are amazing gestures and paths to connection.

SEX FACT

Men consider penis size the third most important feature for a man, while women rate it only ninth.

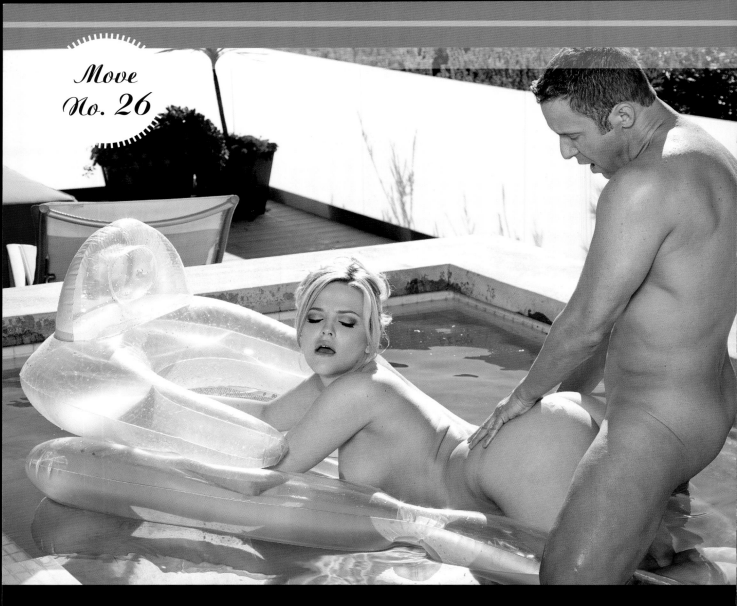

SANDY SHENANIGANS

Sex on a beach is a fantasy for those wanting to get away from it all and get off at the same time. Learn all the tips and techniques for having sex at the beach (or lake) without the sand burns or getting caught, and help your lover fulfill her beach fantasy like a pro, even if you have never had sex on the beach in your life. She will fall for your thoughtfulness and be feeling sexy from sunrise to sunset.

The Move: Sandy Shenanigans

THE PREPARATIONS

★ Scout out a beach or lake that has small waves and isn't that crowded, or that has a secluded area. Choose a school day or night when no little ones are around.

★ Search for some amazing-smelling suntan oil.

★ Pack the following: blanket, beach towels, inflatable raft, sun tent (if you have one), silicone lube, extra towels, wipes, beach music (reggae is great), lots of water, and a picnic cooler filled with piña coladas or her favorite drink, fruit, cheese, crackers, chocolate, and so on.

THE LEAD-IN

Customize and send your own Evite invitation, complete with a favorite beach image and music clip. Have the message read, "Escape with me to the beach tomorrow. I will pick you up at 11 a.m. Bring a bikini."

THE FOREPLAY

① Once you've arrived at the beach, strip down to your bathing suit, lay down the blanket, inflate the raft, play the music, and pour the drinks.

② Pull out the suntan oil and offer to rub it on her back. Have her lie down on her belly. Move her hair aside and generously apply the oil. Start at her back and work your way down, giving long, broad strokes. Sit to one side of her at her ankles and slowly move your hand up her sun-kissed legs while your thumb lingers on her inner thigh. Have each upstroke get closer and closer to her bikini line, ultimately sliding a few fingers underneath her bathing suit.

③ Move so you are situated to one side of her bottom and closer to her back. Begin applying suntan oil by going around the bathing suit strings, but eventually untie or unhook her top. Give her broad strokes that extend to her armpit and the fleshy part of her breast. Repeat the stroke, massaging the oil into her breast and getting closer and closer to her nipple.

||||||||||||||||||||||||||||||||||||||||||||||||||||||||||||||||||||||||||||||||||||||||||||||||||||||

SEX FACT

Twenty-six percent of participants in the 2005 Durex Global Sex Survey reported that they have had sex on the beach.

★ The Main Act

1. Ask her to join you in the water. Grab the raft and the silicone lube. Tell her to lie face up, floating on the raft, and scoot down so her legs are hanging off the edge.

2. Send shivers down her spine by kissing her sun-splashed shoulders and neck while she floats in the water.

3. Position yourself between her legs. Discreetly trace a finger up to her erect nipple. Reach farther down, under her bathing suit (or on the outside), and gently rub her clit back and forth as you look in her eyes, kissing her and feeling her waves of desire.

4. If you can, turn your back discreetly to the shore, push her bathing suit aside and dive your tongue between her labia. Ride your way to the cliffs of her clit, moving your tongue up and down and side by side as you taste the salt of her seas.

5. Kiss your way back up to her lips so you are face to face and she can smell her essence on your face.

6. Keep her on edge. There's more.

7. Bring the raft to waist-high water.

8. Lower the raft, pull her close, pull out your penis, put on the silicone lube, and enter her.

9. Lift her rear and pull her in for deeper penetration.

10. Lean over her and pull the raft to and away from you, riding the waves all the way to climax.

11. When the winter snow and rain begin to fall, warm your hearts with a beach day in your living room. Play your reggae music, pour some piña coladas, and don't forget the suntan (or massage) oil.

RELATED MOVES

★ Position her on her belly for rear entry. This also provides deeper penetration.

★ Lie on the raft together and enter her side by side. This is perfect for intimacy but more challenging for balance; however, you can have a lot of fun trying.

★ Set up the sun tent and have sex inside. Take a nap, wake up, and do it again.

♀ WHY IT WORKS FOR HER

★ She can enjoy the view, the romantic fantasy, and your cock all at the same time.

★ Positioning her legs differently gives her different sensations inside her vagina and provides some friction from the labia on her clit. It is particularly sensational in positions such as this where she is in high arousal and anticipation of entry.

♂ WHY IT WORKS FOR HIM

★ This is actually a very satisfying position. When you lift her butt, you are in control of where the sensations hit your cock.

★ The combination of warm sun, cool water, and the slipping and sliding on your penis really can't be beat.

★ If you love the ocean and outdoors, this is a natural and easy way to express your romantic side.

||||||||||||||||||||||||||||||||||||||||||||||||||||||||||||||||||||||||||||||||||||||||||||||||||||||||||||||||||||

THE SEXPERT SAYS

The goal is to have more positive experiences in your memory bank than negative ones. A new sexual adventure such as Sandy Shenanigans can give you a surplus of positive memories. When the going gets tough, that's what you want.

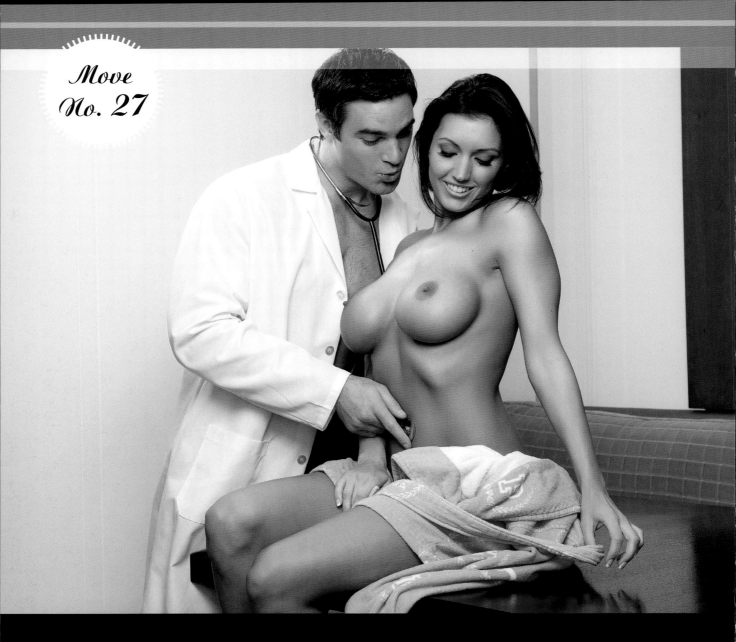

THE MEDICINE MAN

Sex (and orgasm) releases some of the best natural drugs on the planet. In this scene you will use your own line of sexual medicine to heal yourself and your lover. With her on her back, give her your cure-all, an oral orgasm that will alleviate all her pain. Chances are she will be back for more regular and frequent visits, demanding to see the doctor!

The Move: The Medicine Man

THE PREPARATIONS

★ Know the power and medicinal benefits of orgasm. Practice orgasmic medicine on yourself and reach for an orgasm before reaching for the prescription. Record the many ways you can use orgasm. Here is a short list: anxiety, insomnia, fatigue, muscle ache, and headache. It's even good for overeating (what are you really hungry for?).

★ Have a white jacket?

★ On a piece of paper, write "Dr. Cummings" and tape it to the door.

THE LEAD-IN

There are several ways you can lead into this. For example:

Seek the opportunity. The next time she talks about a simple ailment such as a headache, muscle ache, or sore throat, tell her you want to help. Kiss her forehead and tell her that the doctor thinks she has a fever, but that you can't be too sure without the full exam.

Leave her a reminder note that she has an appointment with the doctor: "You have an appointment with Dr. Cummings for an exam at his office on _____ at _____ ."

THE FOREPLAY

① Hand her a robe, ask her to undress, and invite her to come sit on your exam table.

② Open her robe, put your hand over her heart, and listen to her heartbeat; give the usual doctor "hmmm, ahhh." On your way out of her robe, brush your fingertips over her nipples.

③ Brush your hand down to her waist and explain that you need to do a pelvic exam. Have her bend her knees and slide down to the edge of the table so her ankles are to her bum.

④ Do a close examination. Notice the shades of pink and hues of purple. Get close enough so she can feel the warmth of your breath.

⑤ Explain that you are going to apply a topical oral treatment . . . with your mouth. Put your lips around her clitoris as you pucker your lips and suck from base to tip. Tilt your head to the side, look up at her, and feather your tongue over the clitoral glans. Luckily for her, you are the only doctor that specializes in this kind of treatment and she already has the appointment.

||||||||||||||||||||||||||||||||||||||||||||||||||||||||||||||||||||||||||||||||||||||||||||||||||||||||||||||||||||

SEX FACT

Many women find that an orgasm's release of hormones and muscle contractions help relieve the pain of menstrual cramps and raise pain tolerance in general. (It's preventive medicine, too.)

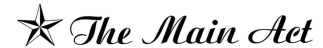# The Main Act

1 Have her lie down on the exam table, face up. You stand at the edge of the table, which should be about 12 inches (30.5 cm) below your penis.

2 Raise her legs and rest them on your shoulders. Lift her pelvis so it is tilting upward and her back forms a straight line to where penis and vulva meet.

3 Place your hands under her hips so you can hold her at the ideal angle for thrusting.

4 Spread your legs open to adjust the height and align with her. Tell her, "I am going to insert deeply and I want you to relax. So far, you are responding well to this treatment."

5 Ask her to flex her PC muscle so you can feel the tightness on your cock.

6 She can use her arms to brace herself up. Continue to hold your hands under her hips and keep her bum up at just the right angle while you ease her pressure and orgasm her pain away.

7 Climb onto the table or bed and wrap your arms around her throughout resolution. Invite her back for her next visit.

8 The next time she wakes with a stuffy nose, nip it in the bud by leaving a reminder note for her next visit.

RELATED MOVES

★ For a more complete treatment, get all the angles—rotate her on her sides and stomach.

★ Place her on her side and bend one of her knees and bring it to your chest while the other leg extends over the table. Your penis will access angles and relieve tension she didn't know she had.

★ You can do a reversal with her lying on her chest and her butt in the air, except you likely will have with put her legs under your arms and not over the shoulders. It is a little more effort for you, but the penetration feels nice and the position puts pressure on her clit.

★ For back pains and general stiffness, choose an effortless treatment such as the mouth-to-vulva oral treatment. Put her on the edge of the bed and give her a dose of orgasmic relief.

|||||||||||||||||||||||||||||||||||||||||||||||||||||||||||||||||||||||||||||||||||||||||||||||||||||||||||||||||

SEX FACT

Many women find that an orgasm's release of hormones and muscle contractions help relieve the pain of menstrual cramps and raise pain tolerance in general. (It's preventive medicine, too.). And studies have shown that men who have at least three orgasms per week are 50 percent less likely to die of heart disease. (Shouldn't we all be getting lower health insurance rates if we are having more frequent orgasms?)

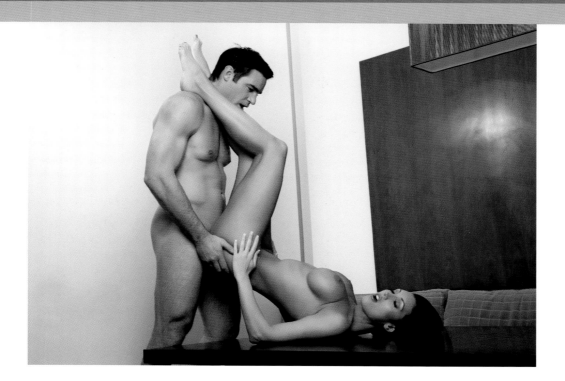

♀ WHY IT WORKS FOR HER

★ The pelvic tilt provides full access to her vagina. It also builds tension for a more intense orgasmic release. Just what the doctor ordered.

★ She will never forget her pelvic exam and how much you care about her well-being. It will put her in touch with her own healing powers.

♂ WHY IT WORKS FOR HIM

★ Easy entrance without a lot of energy commitment means that you can give this treatment all in one visit.

★ You get to be her medicine man, the one with the magic touch, the one who turns sickness into health.

||||||||||||||||||||||||||||||||||||||||||||||||||||||||||||||||||||||||||||||||||||||||||||||||||||||||||||||

THE SEXPERT SAYS

Taoists understand the importance sex has on health. They believe that the genitals correspond with other parts of the body, much like the reflexology points on the foot. Taoists suggest that lovers stimulate the entire penis and vagina because of the added health benefits, and that's easy with positions such as this. Don't ignore the significance of sex on your physical, emotional, and spiritual health.

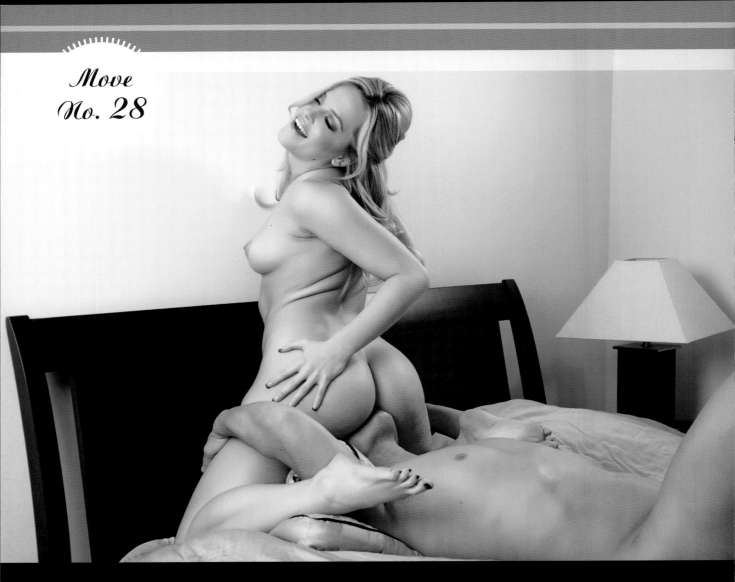

XTRA MILEAGE

She wants you to make love to her for a looooong, looooong time. Experience the positions that work well for you to last longer and possibly come again. Just when you find your favorite position, you will learn more. Knowing a variety of skills and techniques is important so you can be in the moment and confident of yourself as a lover. Xtra Mileage gives you that.

In this move, you will learn how to orgasm without ejaculating so your cock stays hard and you are able to enjoy and share the pleasures of intercourse longer.

The Move: Xtra Mileage

THE PREPARATIONS

★ The first step to being a multiple man is knowing that orgasm and ejaculation are different and can be separated. Orgasm is the contraction and release of tension in the muscles. Ejaculation is a reflex, or an involuntary muscle spasm, that occurs at the base of the spine and results in an ejaculation of fluid.

★ Strengthening your PC muscle is critical to becoming multiorgasmic. Two to 3 inches (5 to 7.5 cm) of the penis is rooted in the PC muscle. Strengthening this muscle is *very* important to stronger erections, more intense orgasm, and better control.

★ Your PC muscle surrounds your prostate, which is the gland the semen passes through. Ultimately, this is the most important step in ejaculatory control. You want to squeeze your PC muscle, which squeezes your prostate, which will allow you to enjoy your orgasm but know when to contract and stop the expulsion of ejaculation.

★ You will want to practice before trying this with your lover so you can be more focused on your own process. To do this, start by masturbating using the following sequence:

1. Breathe deeply. Sit up straight, place your hand on your abdomen, and breathe in through your nose, filling your belly with air so it expands. On the exhalation, your abdomen should flatten.

2. Begin to masturbate. Pay attention to your sexual response cycle. Imagine that resting is at 0 and ejaculation is at 10.0. You want to stop sensation to your penis while you are in high arousal (about a 7.0 or 8.0; long before the point of no return) and gently contract the PC muscle around your prostate.

3. Resume pleasuring yourself, coming closer and closer to the point of no return with each start/stop (9.2, 9.4, 9.6, 9.8, and so on).

4. At 10.0, allow yourself to enjoy the contractions of orgasm in your prostate and sphincter without ejaculating.

THE LEAD-IN

Tell her that you are reading and practicing multiple orgasms and you want to try it with her. Ask for her help in ceasing sensation (stop movement on your penis) when you become close to the point of no return.

||||||||||||||||||||||||||||||||||||||||||||||||||||||||||||||||||||||||||||||||||||||||||||||||||||||||||||||||||||||||||||||||||||||||||

SEX FACT

In his book *Sexual Behavior in the Human Male*, Alfred Kinsey reported that the average number of orgasm for a preadolescent boy was 3.72, only 6.28 minutes apart. Did you orgasm without ejaculation as a boy?

THE FOREPLAY

① One of the best techniques for ejaculatory control is to manage anxieties that lead to performance anxiety and ultimately early ejaculation.

② Be in the moment, put your attention on her, and give her lots of foreplay (maybe even to orgasm).

③ Lie down on the bed with your head at the headboard. Have her sit on your face; this allows her to lean forward, hold on to the headboard, and position herself where she wants to get a licking.

④ Take advantage of the view and really get into the moment. Feel your lips against her soft skin, smell her musk, feel her warmth, and taste her essence. Be so in the moment that you are feeling your cock getting hard giving her oral sex; be so in the moment that you could feel her pussy licking you back. Being in the moment is the trademark of a great lover and is also used to manage early ejaculation. Reach up and roll her nipples between your fingers and stroke your cock with your other hand.

⑤ When you are both ready, have her move into the most comfortable, she's-on-top, face-to-face position for her. Before she does, insert a finger deep inside, rubbing on her cervix and moving the moisture around her entire vulva. Studies have shown that women whose cervix is stimulated become lubricated even when they don't report being aroused.

||||||||||||||||||||||||||||||||||||||||||||||||||||||||||||||||||||||||||||||||||||||||||||||||||||||||||||||||||||

SEX FACT

According to a survey by MSNBC/*Elle* magazine, 41 percent of men say they wish the duration of sex were longer.

||||||||||||||||||||||||||||||||||||||||||||||||||||||||||||||||||||||||||||||||||||||||||||||||||||||||||||||||||||

SEX FACT

Ejaculation occurs about 2 seconds after orgasm at a freeway speed of 70 mph.

||||||||||||||||||||||||||||||||||||||||||||||||||||||||||||||||||||||||||||||||||||||||||||||||||||||||||||||||||||

THE SEXPERT SAYS

Ejaculation is important to prostate health. I encourage men to learn to control ejaculation so that they can manage their energies and last longer if they choose. This position is a good place to start for men with early ejaculation (EE). Causes of EE can include, but are not limited to, masturbation style, shyness, infrequent sex, performance anxiety, or a hurried personality. If you suffer from EE you can also try using a cock ring, numbing agents, or medical intervention.

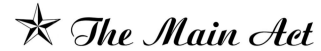

The Main Act

1 Let her do what feels good to her from the woman-on-top position.

2 Stop at 7.0 or 8.0 as you did in practice and redirect your attention to stimulating her orally or digitally.

3 The woman-on-top position is great for stroking the G-spot, which usually involves shallow thrusts. Shallow thrusts don't stimulate the penis the way longer thrusts do, which is another reason that this position is so great for multiple Os.

4 As you get close to the point of no return, lift up her hips or hold them down and ask her to stop.

5 Breathe deeply and fully as you contract the PC muscle around your prostate. You might want to reach around and put your finger on your prostate to centralize and feel the contractions.

6 Resume the stop and start while enjoying the contractions of orgasm without ejaculation.

RELATED MOVES

★ As a general rule, men expend more energy with an orgasm than women do. For this reason, some men choose not to ejaculate at every sex session. Here are a few techniques to help decrease your urge to ejaculate. They focus the attention and interrupt the reflex to ejaculate.

1. Gently tug on the balls. The testicles will naturally rise prior to ejaculation, but gently tugging will help prolong ejaculation.

2. Press on the perineum. While in training for multiple Os, this is the best technique to use during lovemaking because you (or she) can reach back and press on the perineum (before the anus, at the root of the penis).

3. Press your thumb just below the head of the penis. This will help cease sensation so you can clear your head and reset.

♀ WHY IT WORKS FOR HER

★ This position will increase your lovemaking duration and hence her penetrating pleasures.

♂ WHY IT WORKS FOR HIM

★ You can use any position for multiple orgasms. What is most important is mastering the awareness, which means lots of masturbation practice. However, most men find the woman-on-top position best for multiple orgasms and lasting longer because energy is drawn away from the penis, and you can relax and pay attention to your arousal rate while stimulating her nipples and holding her hips if necessary.

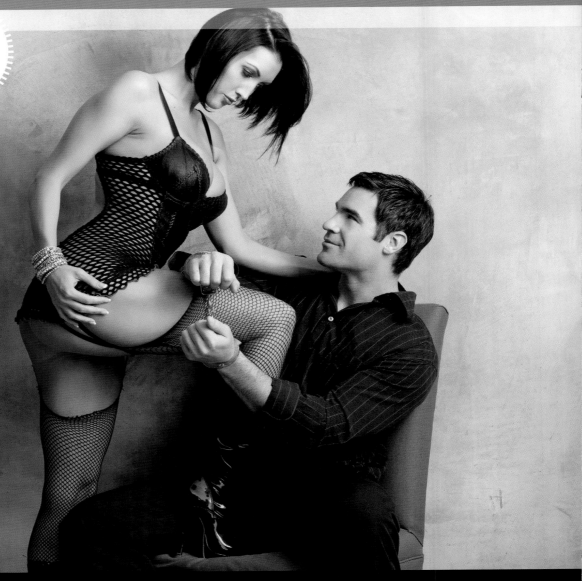

 # DAY AT THE IMPROV

Women love to get "dressed up," and this scenario gives her a lot of that. She has 7 minutes to get dressed, get into character (e.g., saloon girl, police officer, bank robber, sexy superhero, school girl, etc.), and get on your home stage. When she comes out, you seduce her character with your improv sex moves.

The Move: Day at the Improv

THE PREPARATIONS

★ Have a kitchen timer close by.

★ Senses are always more heightened in front of an audience, so set up the camcorder on a tripod.

★ Rent and watch some of your favorite improv.

★ Write each of the following on one side of a note card:

— Two dogs in a park

— Tantric couple

— Superhero and damsel in distress

— Prostitute and patron

— Patron of a gigolo

— Saloon girl

— Schoolteacher and student

— Master and sex slave

— Strangers on the street

— Doctor and patient

— Police officer and bad guy/girl

— Stripper/exotic dancer and customer

— Your own fantasy

— Your girl's fantasy

The Rules

★ She picks a card and does not show you.

★ She has 7 minutes to get ready. Set the timer or play songs you both know and love that are about 7 minutes long. A big part of the fun is getting dressed up. Give her a 90-second warning.

★ When she comes out, you have 10 minutes to enjoy getting to the point of sex. No matter where you are in the process of sexy arousal, you must stop after 10 minutes. This will keep the buildup at an all-time high.

★ Use your imagination. Regular household objects make great props. For example, string licorice makes for fun police handcuffs and whips to be used on the sex slave, the eraser on a teacher's pencil feels nice on the nipples, the smooth coolness of the saloon girl's bottle feels sobering between the thighs.

THE LEAD-IN

Create a program from the list above, print it out, and include the rules along with the date and time of when the show begins. Roll it up, wrap a bow around it, and leave it in the bathroom for her to find.

THE FOREPLAY

①   To get warmed up, you will want to do some sexy improvisation exercises.

②   Stand up straight and, using only your facial expressions, look at each other lustfully. Walk to each other and communicate your lust in a kiss.

③   Do nothing except kiss. Be close with your lips almost touching and your eyes closed, and gently graze the surface of your lover's mouth as you kiss. Get lost in the kiss. If your mind wanders, bring it back and feel the sensations in your lips, and be in the present moment.

★ *The Main Act*

1   Press "play" on the camcorder and set the timer for 7 minutes for her to get ready.

2   When she comes out, react to what is being communicated in dress, words, or gestures. Agree on the scenario, and then build on that. In your mind, say, "Yes, and . . ." as you create a sexy scene. The scene always ends with a sexual seduction of some sort.

3   Accept and go with the first reaction that comes to mind as if it were the best idea you've ever had. Give it all your energy, your enthusiasm, and 100 percent of your emotions as if you had nothing to lose.

4   A shortcut is to think of the role and your end goal of sex. Is your character one of submission, dominance, or equality? Think in terms of these sex equations:

— Face to face sitting or standing = equality

— On top = power

— On the bottom = submission

— Rear-entry insertion = power

— Rear-entry receiving = submission

5   How will you lead in to the position? Do not break character, even if you are the submissive one and she is the dominant one and you are not used to that role. Use your props to up the ante.

6   For fun, try to maintain your role while you are having sex. When the 10 minutes is up, stay in character to end the act.

7 Keep up the sexing sessions, create the buildup, and have an orgasm that's strong enough for an entire cast.

8 Eat popcorn, snuggle, giggle, and watch your sexy improv throughout resolution.

RELATED MOVES

★ I dare you to go out to dinner dressed up as your favorite sexy couple on a day other than Halloween. Go incognito and see whether anyone recognizes you.

♀ WHY IT WORKS FOR HER

★ "Getting ready" can be an arousing part of the overall experience for a woman. Putting a woman in high arousal can make for quicker, multiple, and more intense orgasms.

★ This scenario gives her a chance to get out of her comfort zone and participate in roles she would normally not allow herself to do.

♂ WHY IT WORKS FOR HIM

★ This is a great a twist on typical role-playing games, giving lots of practice in the art of seduction.

★ Different personas mean different techniques and sensations. I dare you to get wild!

||||||||||||||||||||||||||||||||||||||||||||||||||||||||||||||||||||||||||||||||||||||||||||||||||||||||||

SEX FACT

A survey by MSNBC/*Elle* magazine reports that an exciting sex life contributes to sexual satisfaction, which in turn contributes to a satisfying marriage.

||||||||||||||||||||||||||||||||||||||||||||||||||||||||||||||||||||||||||||||||||||||||||||||||||||||||||

THE SEXPERT SAYS

Male clients often tell me that their partners have sex with them, but it doesn't seem like they are really into it. They want to know, "How do I get her to want sex with me the way I want sex with her?" Just when you thought you had arrived with the beautiful home and financial security, she wants more. She wants the seduction and the sincere thought and time of it all.

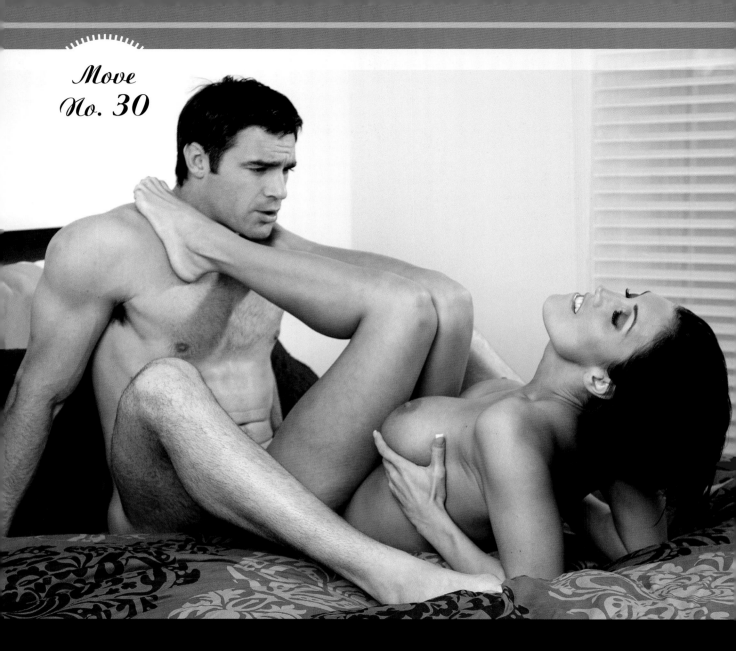

THE GRAND FINALE

This is the Grand Finale, or tour de sex, that you have both been dreaming about. Twenty-four hours

of sex, sleeping, sex, eating, and sex only. No phones, no television, no computers. After full-body

and multiple orgasms, come back to join the world fresh and rejuvenated. Now that's a vacation!

The Move: The Grand Finale

THE PREPARATIONS

★ Make reservations at a hotel.

★ Pack music and candles.

★ Draw a bath right before she arrives.

★ Arrange for her to get away overnight (kids, appointments, etc.).

★ Write the note below.

THE LEAD-IN

Leave a card that says, "Wear the outfit that you modeled for me the other night and meet me at the _____ hotel. See you at 7 p.m."

Tell the front desk that you are expecting her. Prop the door open so she can walk in to find you sitting in the candlelight listening to music and waiting for her.

THE FOREPLAY

① When she comes in, give her your grounding hug, and hold and rock her to the music. Find the beat (revisit Get Jiggy with It), giving her a little bump and grind.

② Lead her to the mirror and have her remove the outfit you got her. Kiss and tease her all over her body as you did in the Kiss of Date.

③ Begin to pleasure yourself and invite her to join in for a bit of mutual masturbation as you did in Sex 101. Pay attention and watch her sexual response for the pace, pressure, and speed of how she likes to be touched.

④ Keep the arousal high and walk her to the bubble bath, where you both get in. Read a few pages from the erotic story you wrote for Bedtime Stories as you soak and stroke.

⑤ Take her to the edge of the bed, lay her on her back, spread her legs, and lick her U-spot, gently brushing your tongue over and around it.

⑥ Now, move your tongue up to the clitoris, which should be more erect. Place your lips around the base and give it a suck as you rub your gums on her commissure.

⑦ Take note of her faster heart rate, rapid breathing, sex flush, and other signs of increased arousal. She is *hot*!

SEX FACT

Most recorded orgasms in an hour: 134 for a woman and 16 for a man. (What can *you* do in 24 hours?)

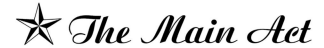
★ The Main Act

1 Lie down on the bed and beg for her to sit on your face so you can taste her and give her a little Oh My Goddess. Let her come on your face. Let's see if she can come again.

2 Have her climb on top and ride your cock for a little Bucking Bronco. The deep G-spot stimulation feels really great even after a clitoral orgasm. Bend her knees and do a reverse cowboy, fucking around the cock doing a 360. Yee haw! (See right.)

3 Remember the techniques you learned from Xtra Mileage. It's okay to shift the center of attention by pleasuring her, stroking, eye gazing, or doing sensual eating. Room service!

4 Stimulate the cervix zone as you did in Blue Pussy. Sit up on the bed in the seated position with your hands behind your back and your knees bent. She is also sitting with her hands behind her, but her ankles are on your shoulders and her butt is in your lap.

5 Blindfold her and lay her down sideways as you did in Pleasure Party and insert a small dildo or plug into her anus. Insert your cock in her vagina and feel how the butt plug narrows the vaginal opening and gives tighter sensations for you.

6 Remove the dildo and penetrate her from behind with your cock. Place the vibrator on her clit. Ask her to tell you when she comes. When she gives the sign, remove the vibe and cease sensation for a two-second count. Reinsert the vibe and watch her pop.

7 Hold, snuggle, and caress her throughout resolution. Repeat. Repeat. Repeat.

♀ WHY IT WORKS FOR HER

★ The hotel room experience offers padded walls so she has the freedom to fully express her orgasms. Isn't that hot?

★ No cooking, cleaning, or work. This is like a mini vacation.

♂ WHY IT WORKS FOR HIM

★ You will have a lot of variety, time, and skill to do it all.

★ You will also enjoy that your lover is more relaxed without the distractions of day-to-day responsibilities.

|||||||||||||||||||||||||||||||||||||||||||||||||||||||||||||||||||||||||||||||||||||||||||||||||||||||

THE SEXPERT SAYS

When you reenter the world, think about how you will restructure your life so you have plenty of time for sex and pleasure. It will only stick if you create the time and protect it. I dare you to have a full 24 hours of only sex, sleeping, sex, eating, and sex every month.

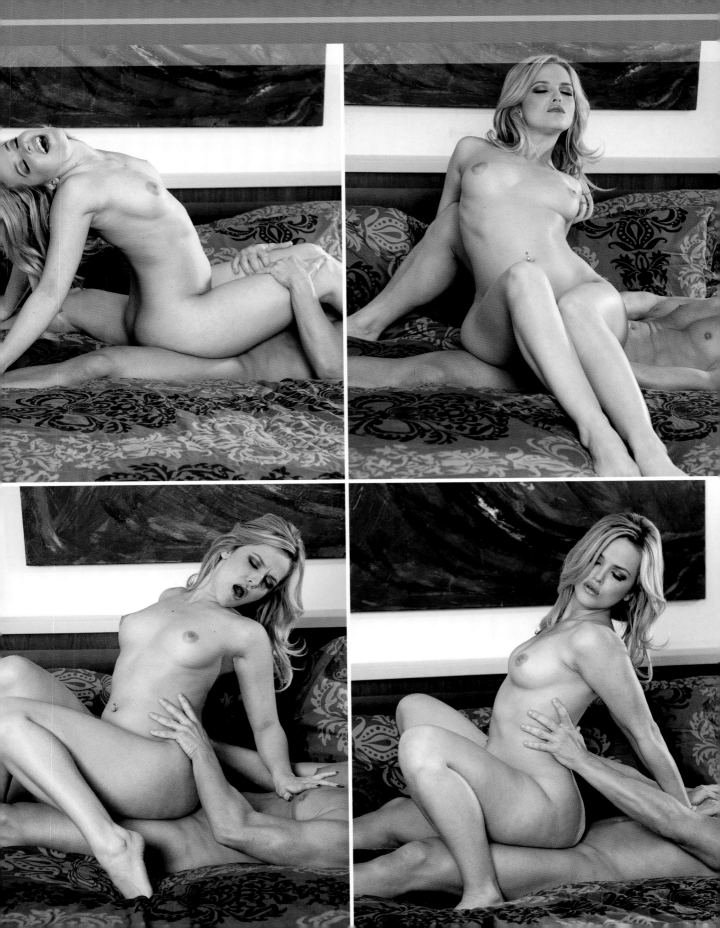

BASIC FEMALE ANATOMY: YOU'VE GOT <u>TO</u> KNOW <u>HER</u> PARTS

You can't expect to drive her crazy unless you know how to drive her car. Here is a breakdown of her erotic parts.

Anatomy 101

The female genitalia are composed of the following parts.

VULVA

A politically and anatomically correct name, the vulva, also known as pussy or yoni, is the external visible female genitalia.

★ **Mons or mons veneris (Latin for "mound of Venus"):** This soft spot on top of the pubic bone is sensitive to the touch and nice for arousal, but stimulation there generally won't bring her to climax.

★ **Labia majora (large outer lips):** The labia majora compose a somewhat sensitive area that overlays and protects the more delicate inner layer of the vulva. The mons and the outer lips are covered with hair (that some women wax or shave). Many women find that removing the hair increases sensitivity to touch.

★ **Labia minora (smaller inner lips):** These inner, more sensitive lips swell and change color when she becomes aroused. They are more slender in size than the outer lips, though they sometimes extend down past them.

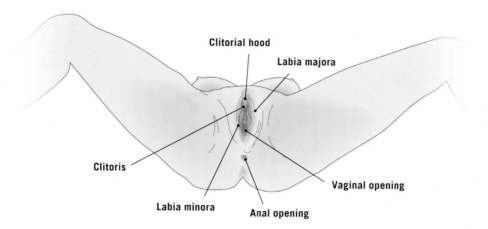

Clitorial hood

Labia majora

Clitoris

Vaginal opening

Labia minora

Anal opening

CLITORIS

The clitoris (slang terms include "the little girl in the boat," "the bean," "the magic button," and "the pearl") is the only organ on either the male or the female body designed solely for pleasure. The clitoris has 8,000 nerve endings and operates within a network of 15,000 nerve endings that service the entire pelvic region. Knowing this should remind you that it would be nearly impossible for her to have an orgasm that is not clitoral in nature.

★ **Clitoral hood:** This little outgrowth or overgrowth of skin covers and protects the clitoral glans. When she becomes aroused, the clitoral glans protrudes from the hood, though in some women, just barely.

★ **Clitoral glans or shaft:** When people refer to the clitoris, they are usually talking about the clitoral glans, or the "knob" of nerves that connects the clitoris to the vagina. What a potent little piece of genital property this is! Learning what your lover likes and dislikes when it comes to stimulating this precious gem is key to her long-term orgasmic happiness.

★ **Crura (a.k.a. wings):** *Crus* translates as "leg," thus *crura* means "legs." Located to the right and left of the urethra, these two internal portions of the clitoris run back to the pubic bone. They are shaped like an upside-down V, connecting to the clitoris at the point of the inverted V.

SEX FACT

The clitoris is developed from the same fetal tissue as the penis.

- ★ **Vestibular or clitoral bulbs:** A string of bulb-shaped aggregations of erectile tissue, the clitoral bulbs extend down beneath the labia minora. When a woman is aroused, they fill with blood, making the vulva swell.

- ★ **Front commissure (external):** The commissure is the smooth area just above the clitoral head and protective hood and just below where the lips (labia majora) meet. A cordlike structure, this area contains nerve fibers that cover the entire clitoral shaft. During intercourse, this area can be stimulated by pressure from the pubic bone; during oral sex by pressure from the upper lip. The commissure can take more intense pressure and is not as highly sensitive as the clitoral glans, making it perfect for clothed foreplay.

- ★ **Fourchette:** Technically translated, *fourchette* means "dessert fork." This is the bottom edge of the lips beneath the vaginal entrance, neighboring the perineum.

VAGINA

The vagina is the elastic, muscular canal connecting the uterus to the outside of the body. When she becomes aroused, the vagina expands in width and length and produces lubrication, though additional lube may be needed.

CERVIX

The cervix is the narrow end of the uterus that connects it with the top of the vagina. It feels hard to the touch and expands with arousal and orgasm.

Some women report that stimulation to the anterior fornix erogenous (AFE) and posterior fornix zones surrounding the cervix offers an intense orgasm and an emotional release. The AFE zone is located about 4 inches (10 cm) beyond the G-spot, toward the front of the cervix, while the posterior fornix is located in the same area but at the back of the cervix. The anterior and posterior fornices have been described as a ringlike structure that encircles the cervix, with the texture similar to that of the back of a Frisbee.

|||||||||||||||||||||||||||||||||||||||||||||||||||||||||||||||||||||||||||||||||||||||||||||||||||||||||||||||||||||||||||||||||

SEX FACT

Any place can be an erogenous zone. Sex researcher Alfred Kinsey found that some women could reach orgasm by having their earlobes nibbled or eyebrows stroked.

G-SPOT

The much-hyped G-spot is a spongy, walnut-size mass of tissue located approximately 1 to 3 inches (2.5 to 7.5 cm) up on the front wall of the vagina. You can feel it by inserting two fingers into the vagina and making the come hither gesture.

URETHRA

Urine exits the body through the urethral opening.

★ **U-spot:** This small mass of erectile tissue above and on either side of the urethral opening is very sensitive to erotic stimulation. This is relatively undiscovered territory for most women (and their lovers!).

BARTHOLIN'S GLANDS

Located slightly below and to the left and right of the vaginal opening, the Bartholin's glands secrete small quantities of lubrication when aroused.

SKENE'S GLANDS

Located behind the rear wall of the vagina and around the lower end of the urethra, the Skene's glands swell with blood during arousal.

ANUS

The exit for the colon, the anus is also very rich in nerve endings. Some women enjoy having their anus stimulated with a finger, a tongue, an anal dildo, or a penis. Both men and women have a sphincter muscle that controls opening and closing the anus and that also contracts at the point of orgasm.

|||||||||||||||||||||||||||||||||||||||||||||||||||||||||||||||||||||||||||||||||||||||||||||||||||||||||||

SEX FACT

The women of Abyssinia were able to straddle a man and bring him to orgasm using the contractions of their PC muscle alone. This practice was also known as *kabazzah*, or "holder." Another word for this practice is *casse-noisette* (nutcracker).

PUBOCOCCYGEAL (PC) MUSCLE

This hammock-like muscle stretches across the floor of the vagina from pubic bone to tailbone; it controls urine flow and contracts during orgasm. If she—and you, because men have it, too—exercise this muscle using Kegels, it will become stronger, enhancing sexual pleasure and intensifying orgasm for both of you. If she has a strong PC muscle, she will be able to "grip" your penis, and even pull it in and out of her vagina.

For women, regular Kegels keep the vagina toned after childbirth and postmenopause. Not only does a strong PC muscle make your orgasm more likely and more intense, but it also facilitates multiple and extended orgasms.

HOW TO FIND HER (AND HIS) PC MUSCLE

Here's how your lover can find her PC muscle: Start by stopping and starting the flow of urine. Once you have located the muscle, begin with a short Kegel sequence.

Contract the muscle 20 times at approximately one squeeze per second. Exhale gently as you tighten only the muscles around your genitals (which includes the anus), not the muscles in your buttocks. Don't bear down when you release. Simply let go. Do two sets of 20 twice a day. Gradually build up to two sets of 75 per day.

Then add a long Kegel sequence. Hold the muscle contraction for a count of three. Relax between contractions. Work up to holding for 10 seconds, then relaxing for 10 seconds. Again, start with two sets of 20 each and build up to 75.

Once you are doing 300 repetitions a day of the combined short and long sequences, you will be ready to add the push-out.

After relaxing the contraction, push down and out gently, as if you were having a bowel movement with your PC muscle. Repeat gently. No bearing down.

Now create Kegel sequences that combine long and short sequences with push-outs. After a month of daily repetitions of 300, you should have a well-developed PC muscle. You can keep it that way simply by doing sets of 150 several times a week.

A Variation for Her: The Kegel Crunch

Vary your Kegel routine by doing them while exercising. For example, do Kegels as you perform pelvic crunches. Contract your PC muscle as you pull in your stomach muscles. Release both at the same time.

A Variation for Him: Add Weight

As your PC muscle grows stronger, you can perform your exercises with first a damp handkerchief, then a facecloth, and finally a hand towel draped over your penis.

Her Sexual Response Cycle

There are general stages of arousal common to all of us, yet specific to each of us. Paying attention to her sexual response cycle and flowing with her moods is the art of lovemaking and what will make you the best lover she has ever had. Women's moods are so intricate that this could be a lifelong practice with the same woman.

SIGNS OF EARLY AROUSAL

★ Her heart rate increases and her blood pressure rises.

★ Her body muscles tense.

★ The vagina begins to lubricate.

★ The nipples and clitoris swell as they become engorged with blood.

APPROACHES

At this stage you want to psychologically and physically engage the female form. The scenarios are a creative way for you to initiate this phase. Approach her with the intention of authentic appreciation, reflecting back her own beauty. Initiate physical contact with the following:

★ Soft kisses

★ Relaxed eye contact

★ Light touches

★ Long, slow strokes

★ Gradual buildup

AS SHE BECOMES MORE AROUSED

★ Breathing deepens, and she may moan or gasp.

★ Muscle tension increases, toes may curl, and spasms might show on the feet, face, and hands.

★ She sweats.

★ As the vagina swells with blood, the genitals appear darker.

★ The clitoris becomes larger.

★ Her breasts may even increase in size to become more full.

★ Her body flushes with a red tone.

APPROACHES

★ Incorporate a rhythm, establishing patterns and sets.

★ Apply pressure.

★ Increase the pace.

★ Apply direct contact to the clitoris and surrounding erogenous spots.

★ Suck various places to direct energy.

★ Create gaps or moments of no stimulation.

★ Be present, watching and listening to what she likes.

★ If performing oral sex, hold on to her as she approaches orgasm.

DURING ORGASM

★ She has muscle contractions and loses control. Depending on the intensity, she may have between three and fifteen contractions occurring at 0.8-second intervals. She may also experience contractions in other parts of her body such as the sphincter.

★ Her body may become rigid at the highest point of orgasm.

★ Some women ejaculate fluid.

★ Sex flush becomes brighter and more noticeable.

APPROACHES

★ Be steady, holding her in place. Maintain contact with her clitoris and stimulating areas.

★ Women do not need to repeat the entire cycle to orgasm again. Once they are in the orgasm phase, they are highly orgasmic.

AFTER (THE LAST) ORGASM (REFRACTORY PHASE)

★ Increased amounts of oxytocin, the "cuddle hormone," are released into the body.

★ The clitoris and nipples become very sensitive.

★ Sex flush disappears.

APPROACHES

The refractory phase is an important part of the experience. Interrupting it would be the same as cutting any of the other phases short. How long should you be in this phase, you ask? Ideally, until she breaks free from your embrace, but 20 minutes is a safe amount of time.

★ Slow down direct stimulation to erogenous zones to a stop.

★ Be present with her.

★ Hold, caress, and celebrate her.

Resources

BOOKS

Carrellas, Barbara. *Urban Tantra: Sacred Sex For The Twenty-First Century.* New York: Random House, 2007. Practical and easy to understand concepts for the urban lover.

Chia, Mantak and Douglas Abrams. *The Multi-Orgasmic Man: How Any Man Can Experience Multiple Orgasms And Dramatically Enhance His Sexual Relationship.* New York: HarperCollins, 1997. A step-by-step guide on being multi-orgasmic and more.

Bakos, Susan Crain. *The New Tantra Simple and Sexy: Longer, Better Lovemaking for Everyone.* Beverly, MA: Quiver Books, 2008. As the name suggests, a simple and sexy book that is rich in ideas and techniques. Like all Quiver books, it's complete with gorgeous pictures.

Kerner, Ian. *She Comes First: The Thinking Man's Guide to Pleasuring a Woman.* New York City: Harper Paperbacks, 2010. A classic book that offers some very important fundamentals that are often overlooked, and more.

WEBSITES

The Happy Endings Company

www.TheHappyEndingsCompany.com
This site includes free downloadable videos, books, and other affordable options for receiving sex coaching on a range of issues.

The Kinsey Institute

www.kinseyinstitute.org
The Kinsey website shares some classic research that is valuable in the understanding of human sexuality to this day.

Society for Human Sexuality

www.sexuality.org
The objective of the Society for Human Sexuality (SHS) is to share sex-positive information over the internet. The site contains information and interviews from leading researchers and sexologists on topics such as safer sex, erotic massage, erotic talk, flirting, the G-spot, swing communities, and poly lifestyles.

About the Author

DR. SONIA BORG is a sex coach, clinical sexologist, best-selling author, speaker, and sex educator. She coaches clients to have their version of the best sex of their lives, both remotely and in person from her office.

Dr. Sonia earned her Ph.D. in human sexuality and masters in public health from The Institute for the Advanced Study of Human Sexuality in San Francisco and her masters degree in communication from San Francisco State University. Sonia is certified as a clinical sexologist by the American College of Sexologists and is a member of the American Association of Sexuality Educators Counselors and Therapists (AASECT).

Sonia has been featured on television and radio shows such as *Discovery Channel Canada*, *Playboy Radio*, *Good Morning San Diego*, and programs on KUSI in San Diego. She is the author of *Oral Sex He'll Never Forget*, *Oral Sex She'll Never Forget*, and *Spectacular Sex Moves He'll Never Forget*.

Acknowledgments

I am blessed to have so many sexy friends and associates who have contributed to helping make this book a reality. It was a true collaboration. Quiver Books, thank you for another amazing opportunity. It has been a sincere pleasure to share a sex positive message one book at a time. Barbara Call, thank you for your patience, insight, and ideas for development. A warm thank you to readers Kim Borg, M. Engal, Jillian Brose Goodger, Nick Karras, and Sayaka Adachi for your fresh, erotic ideas and inspirations.